SIMPLE STEPS TO A BETTER YOU

-An Informative Self Help Guide for Improving the Well Being of Women-

La Lura White, M.D., Pamela Burns, M.A.T.

Copyright © 2013 by La Lura White, M.D., Pamela Burns, M.A.T. All rights reserved. This book or any portion thereof may not be reproduced or used in any manner whatsoever without the express written permission of the publisher except for the use of brief quotations in critical reviews and certain other noncommercial uses permitted by copyright law.

www.secondopinion2.com

Published by SecondOpinion2, Inc.

ISBN 978-0-9893424-0-7

DISCLAIMER

The remedies contained in this book are not intended to be used to diagnose, treat, cure, mitigate or prevent any disease. These remedies and/or recipes have not been clinically proven or evaluated by the FDA. All content, including text, graphics, images and information available are for general informational purposes only. The content is NOT intended to be a substitute for your doctor's or health practitioner's medical advice, diagnosis or treatment. Never disregard professional medical advice, or delay in seeking it, because of something you have read in this book, on our website or affiliated websites. Never rely on information in this book in place of seeking professional medical advice. You are always encouraged to consult with your doctor or healthcare professional with regards to information contained in this book. Please keep in mind that the remedies provided in this SHOULD NOT BE USED IN ISOLATION. It needs to be coupled with a proper diet and a regular exercise program to experience results. Actual results may vary.

TABLE OF CONTENTS

Chapter One - What Are Genes and How Do Your Genes' Fit? ...**1**

Chapter Two - Improving Your Face ...**10**

Chapter Three - Au Natural ...**29**

Chapter Four - Not In The Gym Exercises ...**47**

Chapter Five - Healthy Eating ...**60**

Chapter Six - Dietary Changes For Common Health Problems ...**77**

Chapter Seven- My GYN Exam ...**99**

Chapter Eight- Relationships: Control the Madness ...**116**

Chapter Nine- When Women Are Safe and Unsafe ...**125**

Chapter Ten- Your Finances - The King is in the Counting House ...**142**

Talking To My Friends About Health ...**159**

Appendix ...**170**

About the Authors ...**181**

Bibliography ...**186**

DEDICTATION

This book is dedicated.....to my wonderful children. My daughter, Tasha who has blessed me with three beautiful grandchildren and my son Ryan, a remarkable sports journalist who keeps me centered.

It is also dedicated to all the women I have treated over the last thirty years, who served as my inspiration, by providing me with the ideas that allowed me to choose the topics addressed in this book.

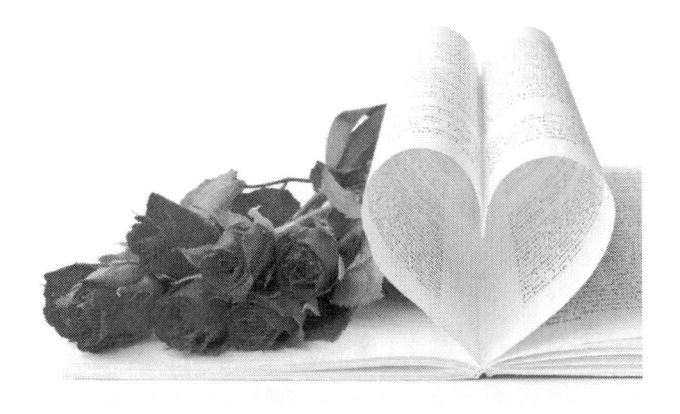

INTRODUCTION

We live in a society where people are obsessed with their personal appearances. Encouraged on a regular basis with tantalizing ads promoting facial creams, teeth whiteners, diet pills, sweatbox exercises, suffocating spandex, cyclic Botox and the ultimate knife-wheeling event, plastic surgery.

Always promising to bring back that youthful appearance to an over gullible audience that has lost the ability to find their true reflection. Baby boomers are becoming older, and in a constant fight to not be dressed in the normal clothes of aging. The younger ones have a mentally convinced, advertised driven ideology that they are already old.

Involuntarily trapped despite the ongoing mentally engaged struggle that "knows better" but unable to escape.

Simple Steps to a Better You" helps bring back a sense of reality. This inspirational, self-help book is practically designed to assist women in improving their lifestyle-- physically, mentally, spiritually and emotionally. Through small but successful changes, women can find personal but untapped roadways that lead to happier lifestyles. This book will not give you a fallacious answer to life's personalized afflictions or unlock a fantasized fountain of youth.

However, it will make you laugh, cry, inspect, explore, investigate and scrutinize. But more importantly, to think about and uncover the many untapped roads you still have left to travel.

Ultimately understanding that it only takes Simple Steps... to get to a better you.

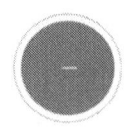

Stop.Go.
How would you know?
Without lights red or green.

Walk.Run.
Will you do either one?
Should the earth beneath you leave?

Cry.Smile.
Do you have a choice?
If no tears fell from your face.

Love.Hate
Can it make a difference?
If you did not wake up today.

CHAPTER ONE
What Are Your Genes and How Do Your 'Genes' Fit?

Genes represent the genetic palette of an individual, where the artist's manipulative brush creates a portrait the mirror reflects. Traversing this palette are tumultuous colors that represent all the imaginable facets of life's creation. Hues collide and impish imaginations congregate upon an amorphous canvas. Thus initiates the personalized beginnings of an "etch a sketch" outline.

Arrays of color, swiftly stroked, prance upon our experiences, with the artist often unable to keep up with nature's muse. They script the landscapes formed by alterations within our meaningful existence, capturing those distortions hurled through time. Sometimes Dorian Grey in nature, our future exists based on our actions of today.

A gracefully intended stroke becomes that familiar nose you habitually powder or those sultry eyes so often used to allure. They also miss-stroke, and form the frowns and wrinkles, cast down by life's emotional tolls. Those unwanted cavernous crevices deeply whittled by heavily trodden pathways, able to capture our essence, a mixed bag of true pleasures and weighted sorrows.

Still, it is within this genetic culprit of pre-destined inheritances that splash our canvas into a self-portrait. Mischievously influenced by nature's spirited hand, our behavioral attitudes and even physical manifestations lead us into becoming constructed. Are we a product of natural selection or a prisoner of rogue mutations?

Our outline begins its initial shape at birth, but later molded by our life experiences and the decisions we make. Decisions we don't understand. We find ourselves often perplexed by that self-image staring back at us from the mirror, and unable to find an acceptable answer to, "Did I do that?"

Despite the fact the answer is "yes", the reasons remain obscured. What transgressed during our life experiences that solidify our present state? Unconsciously manipulated into a thought to be structured lifestyle, which upon second glance, finds you not in control. Instead, spiraling into a "Stepford" routine you've lived in too long, to placate family, friends and job commitments. We find ourselves traveling down roads, not walking but pushed.

After working all day, taking care of kids, cooking dinner, homework, doing a few errands; oh now you want me to do what! Do you really think I have any energy left for sex? If blessed to have a quiet moment we find ourselves asking, "Are we really where we want to be?" We live for a long time not at the controls, even though the button is always available. But at some point in our lives we need to take over the controls. Still responsible for the decisions we make, right, wrong or confusing. However not just reacting to our responsibilities, but looking at the larger picture. Making sure it's one in which the "me" has a definitive place and is not missing.

So, let's examine the genetics that leads us down certain behavioral pathways. For it is in understanding these pesky manipulative traits that we begin to understand why we make the decisions we do, again, and again, and again and again. But remember, genetics only fixes our roads, we make it curve.

The quintessence of our ancestors is lineage-linked from an embryonic behavioral pool that was tried and tribulated by their own convoluted journeys and trampled crossroads.

Randomly cast, their persistent determination for a continued legacy through us is unavoidable. So look deeply into that mirror, and reflect upon those family familiarities, that stare so unmistakably back. Your mom's meddling or grandpa's wit leaves indelible traces within your own personality, maintaining the genetic continuum. But ask yourself, is it genes that predestine how you are living life or just how you jig-sawed them together once in your possession?

What the façade world sees as a productive worker, loving wife and capable mother may be a suffocated soul unable to breathe by the entangling weeds of "give me". Once sucked into near lifelessness, the heart barely beating is still expected at a metronome pace. We become further compromised by the lack of balance between what is given and what is given back. Yet we make no effort to release the person inside who may want to live differently. Our relationships become even more entwined as our existence within them age. Not everyone enjoys "Cougar" status and the associated "perks". Some are left to claw out an existence in a relationship that has long ago faded.

***

Sweetback isn't sweet and Super fly is walking. They all got older but what happened to wiser. There is a similar drive as men age that takes them down a male "menopausal road". They too become victims to nature's mischief that has etched elderly changes into a body once buffed. Now the proverbial yardstick of masculinity is the size of their wallet, expense of their car or penile size after Viagra. Only looking into those wall mirrors that cuts off at the shoulders and frame the face, since pride now limits the reflection they want to see. A little Grecian formula, Botox and failing eyesight might convince them not much has changed. They have become the "man in the facial mirror".

It also doesn't help that scientists from Stanford and the University of California-Santa Barbara report, "Older men chasing younger women contributes to human longevity and the survival of the species." Rod Stewart, David Letterman and Ron Isley have all had babies in their late 50's and 60's. As aging women are falling off the fertility race, men are still running. This gives a macho credence to the fact that the occasionally limp can still pimp.

Carl just slipped in the back door, feeling his twenty-year-old girlfriend was well worth the risk. He creeps up the stairs to avoid the reason he is cheating, his wife. Convinced if she would listen more, talk less and treat him a little better... Well, we all know that's not the only reason. His past twenty years have been riddled with responsibility, support, and maintenance, of others. While somewhere in there his own needs have been closeted, dust-covered and forgotten. Carl needs a diversion. Someone that will make him feel good about himself and who better than a twenty-year old. It won't last, but is it suppose to? Just because you date someone younger doesn't mean you're younger. The age abyss creates a dis-communication because you have so little in common. Also arthritic aches and early evening fatigue will soon compete with youthful spirit and sexual longevity.

And the winner is....

But while Carl's diverting, what about his wife?

"After having 4 kids and gaining 70 pounds, my job is to keep him miserable too," utters Carl's wife confidently to her friend. "I know what you mean. Your job use to be to take all his money but you already got that," girlfriend replies. Older women suffer from, "I got everything but him syndrome." With maturity and time, we have reached many of our goals. Our kids have grown but our personal relationship light dims. Something is lost and we don't know how to get it back. We first become jealous as extra weight, thinning hair and a few wrinkles toys with our own security. Next meanness sets in as the only response we know to hurt. Then finally we explode into vengeance. Here comes the "sugar in the gas tank" or "hot grits". No wonder he chooses someone younger. They are not old enough to be aware of those retributions.

Younger girls are culprits too. Engulfed in the "Sugar Daddy Syndrome" and remember space supratentorial is limited. However, they have recognized the RWB, relationship with benefits.. your money, assets, power, and security. That becomes their attraction and shopping at the mall with your credit card a conquerable mission. But what does that say about a woman who doesn't want to earn those things herself. It used to be, "If you give up the milk he won't want to buy the cow." So, why does he want a cow that has no milk?

Now what does older men dating younger women or a man cheating on his wife have to do with one's genetics? Maybe it's because some of us have gotten the "acceptance" gene. Nonsense excuses for a partner's bad behavior seems to replace common sense, accountability and truth, often with associated self-blame. "If I didn't look at his text messages, I wouldn't have found that sext picture," or "If I didn't come home early, I would not have caught him in bed with my girlfriend." Please!

In fairness, there is a field of study called personality genetics and some authorities believe biological factors may determine personality. But to be a recipient of the acceptance gene means you also exhibit poor self-esteem, lack of confidence, abuse, exploitation, basically a fool -- and you would have better existed as a door mat.

Also genetic inheritability of idiocy can often be traced back. Explore for a minute the women in your family, their relationships and their "acceptability" of their partner's indiscretions. Then look at the outcomes, and if not favorable, this may be a needed and appreciated glimpse into your own future. The good thing is genetics may influence but not fully decide upon a personality expression, meaning one's behavior can be changed.

Nevertheless, to inclusively understand the "why" of our behavior, a necessity for successful change, we have to start at the beginning.

Each month, a woman releases an egg into a sea of emotion, and if met, bumped into or tripped over effectively, conception begins. A remarkable chain reaction initiates, that is concert conducted into the explosive development of rapidly dividing cells on a mission. Obedient formations cultivate everything from your physical traits like eye and hair color, to your idiosyncratic manners and enrapturing personalities. This commixture of blended genes, interprets, develops and creates your tangible self. For these genes are the human blueprints, plans for building the cells, tissues, and organs -- the ethereal anatomy of God's poetic imagination. Nucleic acid called DNA, (deoxyribonucleic acid), a double stranded, helically twisted structure, houses those genes into an informational database of genetic instructions. Very tech-no-co-logical. The DNA is then chain-linked together to form structures called chromosomes. An individual receives a set of chromosomes from each parent, both equally responsible for not just your well-being but also your... being. Within these two sets of chromosomes, each contains 22 pairs of non-sex chromosomes, (autosomes) and one pair of sex chromosomes. It is the sex chromosome pair combination that determines gender, XX for female and XY for males. Ending the lecture on biology and starting the one on life.

Genetics

Jon and I met in a quiet place, on a quiet road while both engulfed in a hectic life-style. Was I attracted to his alluring blue-eyes against that Mediterranean skin or were we both just looking for unattainable peace? Never the less, we hit it off and spent the next few months exclusive. Unexpectedly but accepting, Jon graciously invited me to meet his family the upcoming weekend.

Nervousness, fears and rejection topped my pre-prophesized list of known responses expected from "the new girl" family encounters. I had traveled that roller coaster many times before. After all, if you are at least 30, living in the United States and dating, you have experienced all of the above rejections. But nothing could be further from the truth.

We entered an enormous room, where inside felt like outside. Up close and streaming through a massive bay window was the most picturesque site. We were faced with the magnificence of nature's hand as she drew a line where the sand covered beach and rippling shoreline played. Suddenly, a frail but welcoming voice could be heard, but visually obscured, as she sat with her back to us in a large fanned wicker back chair. Lovingly known as Mom-Mom, because she refused to be called grandmother. A leftover trait from youthful vain, but now, her age-appreciated wisdom enjoyed the comforts of just living.

With statuesque grace, she rose to greet us with a hello genuine. I just smiled for a moment.

There were those beautiful blue eyes against a Mediterranean skin.

How do your genes fit?

Now comes the fun part.

Genetic traits are just fundamental expressions manipulated by your changing environment and social experiences. Are you aggressive or docile, impulsive or restrained?

Let's look at your mother, father, grandmother, grandfather, and their imprinting affect. Since each of your parents contributes a set of chromosomes, you are pre-destined, foreordained or will inescapably resemble either parent, or a combination of both. Genetics are also entropically intermingling and you can also receive those genes ancestral hidden.

Think of those admirable traits you recall about each of these individuals that were passed on to you. These are the traits that give strength and stamina, the huff spa to your character. Now, look at those traits that would make Hannibal's war elephants run back over the Alps and retreat to Carthrage, those Tasmanian traits you also inherited, but may want to give back. These are the traits that you need to work on changing, controlling or possibly hibernating in the deepest caves of your character repertoire.

Some of these traits can and have made you the best possible person.. Smooches. And others, well let's just say... No Smooches.

Alas, the purpose for this book and why you need to keep reading.

We are all a combination of "Smooches and No Smooches" just as a by-product of our inter-mingling existence. No matter how much we are liked, we are hated and no matter how much we are hated we are liked by somebody. But does that translate into us liking ourselves? Balance can only be achieved when you like yourself, psychologically interpreted as demanding respect, accepting responsibility and treating others amicably or politely leaving them alone. Certain part of our "no smooches" psyche often interferes with our achieving balance, and that's the part we have to work on. Identify them one at a time and the list won't be so long, and then make a conscious effort to positively change.

Now our journey towards a better you have already begun. We will continue to take those simple but successful steps, along a serene and tranquil pathway, that challenges your inner self and outer look. Devoid of the stresses of drastic change, that is often not necessary. Our travels attempt to expand your vision of personal change into achievable realities. Often you just need to take the diverse qualities you came into this world with, and fine-tune them to produce attainable goals. You are not trying to be like someone else, just a better you with a foundation already there. The journey starts with being happy with you who is already there - an attitude change. External achievements produce little satisfaction when the internal soul is not rested. Be proud of being where you are in life, even if you still have a little or maybe a long way to go. Find a balance between your past achievements, however unnoticed, and future goals. As long as you realize them, that may be all that's important.

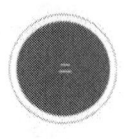

The eyes are the mirrors to the soul
But it's my face that he beholds
For when we walk on a quiet day
It's my smile that takes his breath away

And while I'm basking in this pretty face
Nature comes with her embrace
She draws deep lines where none have been
Cursing me with her aging pen

With dancing glee she marks my face
Wrinkles and crows feet, what a disgrace
Bags grow puffy beneath my eyes
My true age tells, I can no longer lie

So now the true battle begins to task
I'm armed with creams and facial masks
I suck and buzz and stimulate
Soon my facial help can fill a crate

But true success lies within
Eat well and rest is where you begin
Remove the stressors called people we know
Who give your life a hellish glow

Feel good about the person inside
That worked hard and is filled with pride
Who raised the kids and kept the home
And stayed around when hubby roamed

For now it's time to show your pride
Come face to face with the you inside

Once your soul begins to glow
The shine will hide the wrinkles you know

CHAPTER TWO
Improving Your Face

The eyes are the first thing people see when you meet. They reflect a treasure chest filled with your inner glow, personal peace, timed-developed mannerisms and unique personality. However, it doesn't stop there. They also house your cryptic problems, relationship disappointments, internal torments and unveiled crisis. The same encompassing eyes that categorize the true reflection of life's repeated engraving visits also provide roadways into concealed disclosures. All this takes a toll, and your facial appearance becomes a history lesson of an antiquated past.

But not all lessons need to be told. An outward facial glow does wonders for the body, pampers the soul, and should not be conditionally restricted to Tiny Tim's tulip tiptoeing only. Even on a bad day, the face can muster a smile that forks the road you're on and take you to a better place.

When your face looks good, you feel good, so first it is important to know your face.

Within the myriad of facial types and face-specific products there is a niche where you belong. However, it takes a little investigating to understand your face color, skin type and best presentation. The right cosmetics can cleverly transform a blemished outward appearance; but alone, it is not the answer. In addition, lifestyle changes, nutrition, diet and exercise are imperative to improve your overall facial appearance.

What is your skin color?

Blame it on evolution, variations in skin color are considered environmentally adaptive traits passed generationally and genetically over time. Our body hairs decreased to allow for sweating, which provided a more efficient cooling mechanism in hot climates. But stripped of this hirsute protection, the skin was exposed to the harmful UV (ultraviolet) sunrays and their damaging effects. In response, cells called melanocytes, triggered by the enzyme tyrosinase, produced a skin darkening pigment called melanin. This acted as a natural sunscreen, absorbing the harmful sunrays and limiting their ability to penetrate the skin.

The depth of color in one's skin is based on their amount of melanin. Women who are for example of African, Indian, Asian, Hispanic, Arabic and Mediterranean descent has greater amounts of melanin, and therefore can have a spectrum of olive hues and/or darker complexions. There is less risk of developing skin cancer because of the melanin protection, but it is not absolute. If skin cancer does develop, it is usually a more unusual and advanced stage so any concerning skin pigmentations need evaluation. This melanin darkening skin tone also protects Folic acid (Vitamin B9) in the body from being destroyed by sunlight exposure. Folic acid is an important vitamin for many body functions like making and repairing DNA (part of our genetic and nuclear material), cell division and cell growth. However, sunlight triggers the production of Vitamin D, which can be reduced in women with darker skin tones. Vitamin D is necessary to absorb calcium and strengthens our bones. Therefore, women with darker complexions are at greater risk of rickets and osteoporosis (bone-softening diseases).

Caucasian women have less melanin, less sun protection, more penetration of sunrays and greater damage to the DNA (nuclear material) in the cells of their skin and body. This can lead to aging prematurely, cataracts and increased risk of skin cancer. Unprotected, Folic acid (Vitamin B9) and other light sensitive vitamins and minerals can also be damaged by the sunrays, with the potential to increase the risk of low iron (anemia), miscarriages, infertility, neural tube, (birth defects) and affect the immune system and overall health.

Sunrays and Sun-Protectors

It is best to find compatible products that reduce the risk of harmful sunrays all year round, regardless of complexion color, but realizing those with lighter complexions may benefit from more protection.

The sun produces two types of ultraviolet radiation that reaches the earth, UVA rays and UVB rays.

The UVA rays make up 95 percent of the sunrays that penetrate our atmosphere. They are present usually during daylight hours regardless of the time of year. These rays are called long-waves and can pierce the skin deeper, and are more difficult to shield from because they can penetrate glass (like when you are behind the wheel driving) and even our clothes. Because these rays can penetrate into the basal layer of the epidermis or outer covering of skin, they damage skin cells called keratinocytes. It is in this basal area that most skin cancers are found. These rays are also used in tanning beds at strengths up to 12 times that of the sun's rays. Some research suggest tanning before age 30 can increase the risk of melanoma (type of skin cancer) by 75 percent and double or triple the risk of other skin cancers.

The UVB rays are called short waves and do not penetrate the skin's surface as deep as UVA rays. While they are usually more associated with skin reddening and sunburn, due to damage of the epidermis (outer skin layer), they can still cause skin cancers. The strength of UVB rays varies, higher in summer months (April-October) and midday (10am-4pm). These rays are stronger at high altitudes, and can reflect off snow and ice, causing additional damage to the skin.

Sun blocks and Sunscreens:

There is a difference.

Sun blocks provide a barrier or wall between your skin and the sunrays and physically repel or block their penetration. That is because they contain physical or inorganic compounds such as Titanium Dioxide or Zinc Oxide that provide this protection. They are less irritating and may work better for sensitive skin. Although these products reflect the UVB rays, they do not protect against UVA rays.

Sunscreens will chemically absorb and reflect UVB rays, limiting the range of UV light absorbed into the skin. Some products contain Oxybenzone, Titanium Dioxide and Parsol 1789 that can block a small amount of UVA rays and are listed as broad-spectrum protection.

Mexoryl recently approved by the FDA for sunscreen protection may protect you from more of the UVA rays than current sunscreens. L'Oreal (La Roche-Posay) holds the U.S. patent for this product and may be a little more expensive.

It is important to choose the appropriate SPF factor, which is the universal measurement for UVB protection. Those sunscreens with at least a 15 SPF factor block 93 percent of UVB rays while those with SPF of 30 block up to 97 percent. Higher protection can be helpful if one is sun-sensitive or at risk for skin cancer.

SPF refers to the length of skin protection from burning in minutes by the UVB sunrays, and is determined by multiplying the SPF number by 10.

Ex: SPF 15 x 10 minutes = 150 minutes

(time of protection from burning)

Dietary Aids

Healthy Skin: Rosie, Glowing Vibrant

Water:

How many times have I tried to drink the required eight 8oz. glasses of water each day and been successful? None. That doesn't mean to give up hope, just learn a few tricks I am still trying to master. If you can drink the water, that's great, but still read this because I guarantee you have a friend or family member who can't. First commit to have a glass of water in the morning when you wake-up and at bedtime (unless you have problems with going to the bathroom during the night). If you can't do 8 oz., then start with 4 oz.

During the day, try to drink two more glasses of a favorite juice or vitamin water that is half diluted with water. Always check the sugar content, especially if you have Diabetes. You can also add a variety of fruits, herbs and veggies to water like lemons, strawberries, mint, cucumbers, cilantro, oranges and limes to spruce up the flavor naturally. If you can do this for a week, you are on the road to getting more water in your system. Each week, increase your daily intake by one 8oz. glass of water until you reach the goal of eight 8oz. glasses of water each day. Water makes up two thirds of our body weight and is important in flushing out toxins and keeping skin cells hydrated.

Inadequate intake or loss of water can lead to dehydration, tiredness, memory loss, and difficulty concentrating and focusing on small print.

Diet:

Healthy eating with adequate amounts of vitamins, minerals and antioxidants can give your skin a youthful and healthy look so ... Munch, Munch, Munch, Munch, Munch....

Vitamin A is important for healthy skin, hair and bone growth, reproduction, regulating the immune system, vision, especially in dim light, and new cell and tissue growth. There are two types of Vitamin A, depending on whether it comes from an animal or a plant source. Animal sources provide preformed Vitamin A, absorbed in the form of retinol, and can be found in meat, eggs, butter, cheese, cream, liver, kidney and fish oils. However, these can be high in saturated fat and cholesterol. Other foods have been fortified with Vitamin A, like a variety of cereals and milk products. Those fortified low-fat dairy products like low fat yogurt, skim or 2 percent milks may be lower in calories and fat content. Colorful fruits and vegetables contain beta-carotene, a powerful antioxidant that can be converted by the body into Vitamin A. Sources includes carrots, broccoli, kale, mango, papaya, spinach, squash, bell peppers, sweet potatoes, apricots, pumpkin and cantaloupe. The U.S. Recommended Daily Allowance for Vitamin A is roughly 2,000-3,000 IU/day and can vary based on age and gender. This is a fat-soluble vitamin and can be toxic in excess amounts.

Vitamin C helps protect the skin from overexposure to the sun. It reduces the amount of free radical damage that decreases the amount of supporting structures in the skin, like elastic and collagen. It can also stimulate collagen production, reduce wrinkle depth and prevent the oxidative stress that can lead to hyper pigmentation. Excellent sources of Vitamin C include red and green bell peppers, guava, turnips, kale, collard greens and broccoli.

Other Anti-oxidants that protect cells from damage can be found in strawberries, blueberries, blackberries, artichokes, beans (black, red, and pinto), prunes, pecans and plums. They may also provide additional benefits like possible cancer protection, boost our immune and reproductive systems, and help the body absorb calcium for stronger bones.

Healthier oils are labeled cold pressed, expeller processed, or extra virgin. These don't loose important nutrients in processing but limit consumption to 2 tablespoons/day.

Several minerals play a key role in keeping the skin looking healthy. Selenium, an antioxidant mineral, improves skin's elasticity, prevents cell damage by free radicals and may play a role in preventing skin cancer. Good dietary sources are eggs, brown rice, seafood, wheat germ and Brazil nuts. Trace minerals like silica and zinc are important too. Silicia strengthens the body's connective tissue which improves the skin's strength and elasticity. Sources include green and garbanzo beans, asparagus, cucumber, strawberries, mango and celery. Zinc controls the production of oil in the skin and can reduce acne. It also helps the immune system and maintains the senses including taste, smell and vision.

Salmon, Walnuts, Canola Oil, and Flax Seed contain essential fatty acids (EFA) that keep the skin healthy by strengthening the cell membrane's ability to hold water, which helps with skin repair, moisture content, and overall elasticity. The best-known EFAs are omega 3 and omega 6, which must be in balance to have the best effect. Sometimes just balancing these two can result in smoother, younger-looking skin. The body cannot produce its own EFAs. The American diet is abundant in omega 6, which is found in baked foods and grains, but lack in omega 3s, so omega 3 must be increased in the diet. Good sources of omega 3s are cold-water fish like salmon and mackerel, walnuts, flax seed, safflower oil and chia seeds.

Green teas contain antioxidants called catechins. They reduce the amount of free radicals that can damage DNA (nucleic acid) in the body. They have also been shown to fight cancer and reduce the risk of heart disease, stroke, diabetes and dementia.

In addition to a good diet, other helpful activities are:

- Keep digestion normal so toxins can be eliminated.
- Exercise: Good circulation improves oxygen delivery to cells.
- Rest: 6-8 hours each day.
- Avoid the sun between 10 a.m. and 4 p.m. if possible.
- Quit smoking.

Skin Types

- Normal: The skin is soft-textured and well hydrated. There are no visible wrinkles, large pores or lines. There are also no oily or dry areas. The skin has a healthy glow. There may be occasional pimples due to increased hormonal activity, but acne is not a problem.

- Dry: The skin is very fine-textured and velvety. It has an almost "stretched" look, and can be thin and papery because it cannot retain moisture. The skin is very sensitive, and becomes red and parched quickly in the sun or wind. No oily areas are visible. A moisturizer is needed, especially after washing, or the skin feels very tight. Dry skin is especially prone to fine lines, flaking, chapping and cracking.

- Oily: The oil glands in this skin are overactive, and this excess oil gives a coarse texture to the skin with visible large pores. There are no dry areas at all. Oily skin has a greasy shine, dull texture and uneven appearance.

- Sensitive: Skin is dry, flaky and with blushing. Common facial products that can result in burning, tightness, stinging, redness, irritation and/or pustules easily affect it.

- Combination: Both oily and dry or normal areas exist together. There is a T-Zone consisting of the nose, forehead and chin that is oily and dry areas are found around the cheeks, mouth and eyes.

Basic Skin Care Routine

Daily

After cleaning, gently massage facial muscles (especially forehead), eye corners, cheeks and upper chin. Always be careful with skin under the eyes. In this area, you should gently stroke inward to out. This will increase blood flow, promote cell turnover and give your eyes a fresher look. This also helps to tone this area, remove large pores, and prevent blackheads. Always use a moisturizer after cleaning.

Periodic

The term "exfoliate" means to cast off scales, flakes or layers. You should exfoliate your face twice, (2 times) a week to remove dead skin cells and bacteria. Exfoliation allows for new skin cell turnover, and improves skin clarity. You should work around blemishes so they are not irritated during this process.

Cleanser

Normal skin can be cleaned twice a day with a mild soap and warm water. You can also use light to moderate cream cleansers that deep clean without stripping the skin of its natural oils. For occasional breakouts, use an astringent with low alcohol content. This will fight blemish causing bacteria and close pores.

Gently cleanse and massage facial muscles, especially forehead, eye corners, cheeks and upper chin.

Dry skin needs to be cleaned with a cleanser containing an exfoliant that gently removes flaky skin. Cleansers with an oily or creamy base or products that help keep skin hydrated are recommended.

Oily skin needs a cleanser that removes excess oil and maintains moisture on and under the skin's surface. Lathering cream or a bar cleanser works best. These products penetrate the skin allowing for deep cleaning. Be sure your cleanser is oil-free so it will not clog pores.

Combination skin needs a cleanser that will have a balanced formula of both the oily and dry cleansing properties. These cleansers should be rich lathering and have moisture-balancing capabilities.

Toner:

These products are used after cleaning the skin. They can remove excess grime and oils not removed by the cleanser. They freshen and tone the skin, and prepare it for the application of make-up. Toners are pH balanced. The pH determines how acidic or basic a product is. A product rated 7 is neutral, which keeps the skin a little acidy to protect against bacteria. It is important to keep the skin's pH at about 5.5. Toners make your skin feel tingly clean; however, if you have mature, dry, or sensitive skin, you can skip the toner.

Moisturizer:

Apply a daily moisturizer in the morning before applying any makeup. Consider reapplication of the moisturizer throughout the day if your skin is naturally dry. Apply a moisturizer before going to bed at night. Always clean your face before applying a moisturizer.

Natural Toners:

Watermelon Toner
2 tablespoons of fresh watermelon juice
2 tablespoons of distilled water
1 tablespoon of Vodka

Apple Facial Toner
2/3 cup witch hazel
1/3 cup apple vinegar
Several drops aromatic oil

Green Tea facial Toner
2 teaspoons of powdered green tea
1/2 cup of boiling water

1. Let cool and apply
2. Wet with a clean cotton ball and apply with upward strokes.

Natural Cleansers

Lemon and Yogurt Facial Cleanser:
Mix 1 tbsp of lemon juice with 2 tsp of plain yogurt. Apply on face, leave it on for 10 minutes and then rinse with warm water.

Honey Facial Cleanser:

1. Prepare a mixture of 1 tsp of honey, 2 tsp of lemon juice and 1 tsp of yellow sugar. Apply with circular motions, leave on for 5 minutes, rinse with lukewarm water and you're done.

2. Cleanse your face morning and night. With clean hands splash your face with warm water. Place a small amount into a soft washcloth or into the palms of your hands.

Cover all areas of the face and cleanse in a circular motion. Rinse thoroughly with warm water.

Natural Moisturizers

1. Grate one apple and mix with 5 tbsp. of honey. Smooth onto skin, let sit for about 10 minutes. Rinse off with cool water.

2. Mix 1-½ tsps. of Honey, ½ a lemon, 3 tbsp. yogurt and a whipped egg white and apply to face. Let stand for 15 minutes and rinse with lukewarm water.

3. Olive oil, Coconut Oil, Cocoa Butter, Avocado oil, Sesame oil and Beeswax have been used as moisturizers.

4. Use a moisturizer after proper cleaning.

Choosing Cosmetics

Foundations:

It should not match the shade of the skin.

Look for shade cards at the cosmetic counter and use as directed. These are semi-transparent plastic cards that show different foundation shades from light to dark. Hold the card against your jaw or neckline, preferably by a lighted area or window. The color on the card oval disappears against your skin when you have found your right shade. Also ask for tester samples to try before buying foundations. Do not test the foundation against your wrist, as that area is lighter. Dry skin needs a crème or mousse foundation. Oily skin may need a cream to powder or mineral foundation.

Darker Complexion:

Darker skin tones are often naturally elastic, have an oily base, and age slower than fairer skin. As a result, when using facial products, massage oils or creams, you should chose one that is light in texture and less concentrated with oils.

Use a foundation that is creamy, liquid and not oily, but water based, matching the color of your skin (not lighter) and your undertones. Use sparingly, as it can cake on dark skin. Tones also change seasonally; you may need a different foundation in the winter compared to the summer.

Caucasian/Light complexion:

Lighter skin tones are supple but not as elastic as the darker skins. They have less oil. Use a foundation that is oily or has a rich cream bases.

Everyone needs to use products that are sun blocking.

Undertones

Make-up should enhance the undertones of the skin. Yellow or orange tones are called warm undertones, and red or blue tones are cool undertones. What are you?

Take two pieces of cloth, one silver and one gold. Look in the mirror and first place the gold color cloth against your face. If the color of your skin looks brighter against the gold-colored cloth, your skin undertones are warm. Choose foundations that are brown colors like almonds, copper, or honey beige and makeup shades like brown, red, orange, yellow or natural.

Then place the silver color cloth against your face. If your face looks brighter against the silver cloth, your skin undertones are cool. Choose foundations in shades of ivory and pink and makeup in shades of blue, pink, purple, and green.

- If you're blonde, choose cold colors like bluish pink, salmon grey and mauve.

- If you're brunette, choose warm, colors such as powdery plum, chestnut red and amber brown.

For porcelain or milk-and-roses complexions, use transparent, barely-there, make-up to enhance your skin's radiance.

Blushes/Lipsticks

- Fair skin tone: pink or rose.
- Olive skin tone: mauve or berry.
- Fair or ruddy: corals or reds.
- Very dark skin tone: beiges and browns or mauves and berries.

Eye Shadow

- Fair skin: pale or sheer shades, beiges or browns, pinks or rosy colors.
- Olive skin tone: mauves or berries, deep heathers, blues, grays and plum colors.
- Use beiges and browns in moderation.
- Fair and ruddy: corals and reds or pales and sheers.
- Very dark skin tones: mauves and berries, beiges and browns.
- Eyeliners should complement the shade of eye shadow.

- Fair-skinned/Ruddy-toned: brown or brown-black mascara.

- Olive-skinned: brown-black or black mascara.
- Very dark skin: black mascara.

Cosmetic Surgery/Injections
Success vs. failures based on skin color

Cosmetic surgery has become a common and accepted method in today's society to enhance one's beauty. Aside from surgery, there are now medical injections that claim to remove wrinkles and scarring. Although these procedures have been utilized by Caucasians for numerous years, women of color have now begun to embrace these procedures to enhance their looks.

Research on women's skin found that some areas of the faces of women of color have muscular structures that are different than those of Caucasians. Therefore, if you are considering Botox® or Restylane® skin injections for cosmetic reasons, make sure your doctor is familiar with your skin type, and how and where the injections should be made.

There is an increased risk of scarring and keloid formation for people with dark skin. As such, salon treatments should be performed carefully. People of color can get dark spots, discoloration and scarring from an injection. Skin can react negatively to some medical treatments, piercing, plucking, waxing and shaving. These activities make the skin more sensitive, and more prone to side effects. Melanocytes (cells that make the melanin and give the skin its darker tone), can be easily over-stimulated. This can result in reactionary damage, or hyper- pigmentation, that causes patches of skin to become darker in color than the normal surrounding skin. The darker the skin, the more apparent the color variations become.

Skin Stressors

Cigarettes

Aside from the ever-present threat of cancer resulting from smoking cigarettes, research has found that smoking causes additional damage that you don't hear about. A substance in cigarettes called Benzopyrene has been found to seriously deplete the body's supply of Vitamin C.

Vitamin C is vital to the formation of collagen, which are the fibers that make up the support structure of the skin. When the level of collagen is depleted, the skin begins to wrinkle. Research suggests that a smoker's skin ages up to 20 years sooner than that of nonsmokers. Cigarette smoke also contains carbon monoxide, a poisonous gas that can starve cells of oxygen. If you are a smoker, you should be aware of the damage it causes to the skin.

Caffeine

Caffeine is a bitter white alkaloid often derived from tea or coffee, and used in medicine mainly as a mild stimulant. (The American Heritage College Dictionary).

We all know that caffeine is found in our every day diets, as we consume coffee, tea, and carbonated soda drinks. It is also found in cocoa, which is used to make chocolates. What most people may not know are the effects caffeine has on the human body.

Caffeine places a huge burden on the liver as it tries to eliminate toxins from the body. As the acidity levels in the stomach increase; it affects the central nervous system, and increases the heart rate. Caffeine stimulates the brain, giving the illusion of a "rush" of energy. It adds stress to your adrenal glands, increases tiredness, and can contribute to premature skin aging.

There are "high" caffeine drinks like coffee, tea, soda, which many people consume on a daily basis. An average cup of coffee contains approximately 125 mg of caffeine. Tea contains about 70mg, and cola drinks about 55 mg. If you drink four cups of strong coffee a day, you are taking in about 500 mg of caffeine.

In order to cut down on high-caffeine drinks, try decaffeinated coffees and herbal teas as a substitute. This will also increase your water intake.

Sunlight

Did you know that the human body needs sunlight to manufacture Vitamin D? Vitamin D is vital for healthy bones. The mild exposure to the sun from your home environment is sufficient to get the body to manufacture this vitamin. Problems can arise if your skin is overexposed to high levels of intense sunlight.

Overexposure to sun is extremely damaging for lighter complexions, as intense sunlight can cause burning as well as skin cancer. Darker skins, on the other hand, contain much higher levels of pigmentation that protects them from the sun's damaging rays. If you vacation in hot climates, it is vital to use adequate sun protection, especially on the delicate skin of your face.

Poor Diet

Most of the foods sold in this country have been altered by preservatives to allow it to sit in a store for a longer than normal life. Concerns about weight and cholesterol have led many to try to eat healthier. Foods with the label "low fat" have become common in the markets, as consumers believe that these foods will allow them to enjoy their favorite foods, and consume only half the normal amount of fat.

Most people who consume a diet containing low fat products are unaware that they may be depriving the body of some of the fats it really needs. This may sound strange, because we are told to stay away from fats. In this section we will discuss the difference between saturated fats and unsaturated fats.

You may have heard that it is not good for the overall health of the body to consume large quantities of red meat. Red meats are full of saturated fats, which can lead to clogging of the arteries. Red meats also break down into products that are stored in the joints and may cause arthritis. Red meats are harsher on the digestive system, and more difficult to break down than fish or chicken.

On the other hand, unsaturated fats, such as those found in olive oil, are not only beneficial to our health but can also improve the texture and suppleness of skin and hair. Your diet should therefore include minimum amounts of saturated fats and higher amounts of unsaturated fats.

We are a generation of consumers of "processed foods". Potato chips and cookies are often high in salt and sugar and are unlikely to have much nutritional value for the skin. These items should be avoided. By contrast, fresh fruit and vegetables are vital to good skin health and should be eaten as often as possible.

Working on the inside allows you to shine on the outside.

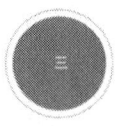

Cleopatra ruled the Egyptian sands
Her beauty mystified
Kept Marc Antony in her bed
And Caesar hypnotized

Nefertiti's eyes entranced
All who looked upon
She bewitched God himself
To sculpt the perfect one

Helen of Troy's exquisiteness
Many suitors did adore
Her face launched a thousand ships
And began the Trojan War

Bathsheba easily seduced
King David to kill her spouse
Then turned his lion's vicious roar
Into a captive mouse

What was their secret ecliptic hold?
On those within their grasp
Unfortunately too much time has gone
And there's no one left to ask

CHAPTER THREE
Au Natural

Many natural remedies are so close, at our fingertips and even in our kitchen cabinets. We just need to know how to put them together, to enhance our "natural beauty". Our ancient glamorous predecessors knew those secrets, found ethereal ingredients and avoided the harsh chemicals and irritants of today's beauty products.

Becoming privy to their natural secrets can enhance our own outer beauty. In addition, you can save money too. So let's take a few tips from those known for their ecstatic beauty. They knew what to do, and now so can you.

Remember, even natural products can have side effects. If you have any health or medical conditions, always first consult your health care provider before using any of the below products or recipes. Also test a small amount on skin first to check for allergies before applying to a larger area. Individual results may vary.

Egyptian Secrets

Various scented and non-scented oils were abundant in Ancient Egypt and served as skin softeners, moisturizers and firming agents. These included Aloe Vera, olive, almond, frankincense, myrrh, and fir oils. Any of these oils can be added to the bath or used as skin oils or moisturizers.

Milk and honey added to Queen Cleopatra's bath was reported to maintain her silken skin. Milk contains lactic acid that can gently slough off dead skin cells. Honey acts as a moisturizer.

I. Bath Therapy:

(Reduces stress, fatigue and the signs of aging. Can also act as a skin rejuvenator.)

Various Bath Oil Regimens:

Milk and honey baths have been popular for centuries. Milk contains alpha hydroxy acids that exfoliate cells and dead skin. Milk proteins improve skin's structure and texture. Though whole, goat or powdered milk can be used, goat's milk is best because it is the only milk that contains capric-capryllic triglyceride, which helps to moisturize and soften skin. Honey is a humectant, meaning it can attract and maintain water which keeps the skin stay well hydrated.

1. Add 2 cups of milk and 2 tbsp. honey to a warm bath. Soak for at least 20 minutes.

2. Pour one tsp. of almond oil or Aloe Vera into a cup of water and leisurely pour it over your body. Exit the bath and pat dry.

3. Add 1-2 cups of Dead Sea salt or other mineral based bath salts to bath water.

You can colorfully decorate the bath water with flowers like Jasmine, Gardenia, Hibiscus, Magnolia, and/or Rose for aromatherapy.

It is told that Queen Cleopatra traveled to the Dead Sea, since it was well known that it contains clay and minerals, useful for beauty and medicinal products.

Do you know Queen Cleopatra?

1. Wasn't an Egyptian, but was of Macedonian Greek origin. She was a descendant of Ptolemy I, a Greek General of Alexander the Great who, upon his death, became the king of Egypt.

2. She was the only person in the entire Ptolemaic dynasty who could speak Egyptian. In addition she was a master of 9 languages.

3. She married her 12 year old brother Ptolemy XIII, when she was 18. They ruled together for 4 years before he was drowned.

4. She had herself rolled up in a carpet and ordered her soldiers to take her inside Ptolemy's palace where Julius Caesar was staying. She did it because she wanted to seduce Caesar, so that he would make her queen of Egypt again.

5. She had 4 children - Caesarion, also known as Ptolemy Caesar (son of Julius Caesar), Alexander Helios, Cleopatra Selene II, and Ptolemy Philadelphus.

6. Mark Antony committed suicide on the battlefield after being misinformed about the death of Cleopatra.

7. Shattered after hearing the news of the death of Mark Antony, she committed suicide by making an asp, an Egyptian cobra, bite her in the breast. She believed, she was the daughter of Egyptian goddess Isis, and the bite of an asp would take her to the gods.

Body Scrubs

#1

1. Mix ¼ cup of honey, baking soda and bath salts together.
2. Add a drop of frankincense, myrrh, Aloe Vera or olive oil.
3. Grind to a paste and rub over the body.
4. Scrub gently with a loofah.
5. Relax for a few minutes then rinse.

#2

1. Mix together 2 cups of sugar, a handful of chopped mint leaves and ½ cup almond oil.
2. Massage over skin and scrub with loofa.
3. Rinse well in tub or shower.
4. Keep scrub in airtight jar for up to one month.

II. Facial treatments:

(Cleans, smoothes skin, reduces wrinkles and eye puffiness.)

Facial Cleansers and Scrubs:

#1

1. Use equal parts of honey and baking soda.
2. Add a pinch of Dead Sea or mineral based sea salt.
3. Rub gently all over face.
4. Rinse well.
5. Can be used also as a body scrub.

(Natron was a hydrated soda ash found in lakebeds in Ancient Egypt. It was replaced with baking soda in this recipe)

#2

1. Mix equal amounts of olive oil and water.
2. Wash face.
3. Rinse well.

Facial moisturizers (should be used after cleansing)

#1

1. Mix 1 tsp sweet almond oil and 2 drops of Frankincense (or 1 drop Frankincense and 1 drop myrrh) essential oil.

2. Gently massage into face and neck at bedtime.
3. Rinse in the morning.

#2

1. Mix small amount of rose or sandalwood oils with equal amounts of almond oil.
2. Apply to face.

#3

1. Mix 1 tbsp. honey and 1tbsp. cream.
2. Apply to face.
3. Wash off after 3-5 min.

Wrinkle Removers

#1

1. Add a few drops of frankincense oil to olive or sweet almond oil.
2. Apply to face and under eyes to reduce wrinkles.

#2

1. Avocado slices can be placed over closed eyes for 20 minutes to reduce eye puffiness and swelling.

#3

1. Balanos, Behen or Almond oil can be applied to prevent dry skin and aging.

Facial Mask

#1

1. Mix equal parts sandalwood and turmeric powder.

2. Add milk and stir to make a paste.
3. Apply to face.
4. Wash off after 3-5 min.

#2

1. Blend equal parts of sandalwood, rose, and frankincense oils.
2. Stir in ¼ cup yogurt.
3. Apply to face.
4. Leave on 5-10 minutes.
5. Rinse well.

#3

1. Apply small amounts of almond oil as an under-eye cream to reduce crows-feet.

III. Hair Treatments (makes hair smooth, silky and reduces thinning)

Hair Conditioners: (should cover with a plastic cap after applying conditioner)

#1

1. Mix equal amounts of almond and coconut oil.
2. Apply to hair for one hour.
3. Rinse well.

#2

1. Use coconut milk or mix equal parts of honey, olive oil, Aloe Vera or limejuice.
2. Let sit for one hour.
3. Rinse completely.

#3

1. Crushed or boiled Fenugreek seeds applied to the scalp were used in ancient times. It was found to restore the hair shaft, reduce hair thinning and promote hair growth.

#4

1. Mix one tsp. Sweet Almond Oil and one tsp. Castor Oil together.

2. Add 10 Drops Essential Oil of Fir Needle or Essential Oil of Rosemary.

3. Mix with your fingers.
4. Rub vigorously into your scalp, especially on areas where hair is thinning.

IV. Oils used as Perfumes:

Just dab a little behind the ears and your inner wrist.

Lavender, thyme, marjoram, chamomile, peppermint, rosemary, cedar, rose, Aloe Vera, olive oil, sesame lily, myrrh and almond oil.

Ancient Egyptian women's attractiveness completed their feminism.

Cassius Dio described Cleopatra:

"For she was a woman of surpassing beauty, and at that time, when she was in the prime of her youth, she was most striking; she also possessed a most charming voice and knowledge of how to make herself agreeable to everyone. Being brilliant to look upon and to listen to, with the power to subjugate every one..."

Indian Secrets

Facial Creams and Moisturizers:

#1

1. Grate raw coconut.
2. Remove the milk.
3. Apply to face and lips.

#2

1. Combine 1 tbsp orange juice, 1 tbsp. lemon juice and 1 cup of yogurt (increasing liquid ingredients can make the cream thinner and smoother).
2. Make into a paste.
3. Apply as a mask.
4. Leave on for 15 minutes and wash off.
5. Apply to face as a moisturizer.

#3

1. Combine 1 tsp. of honey with a small pinch of turmeric powder (using too much can stain the skin).
2. Mix into a paste.
3. Smooth over your face.
4. Let it sit for 15 minutes.
5. Rinse thoroughly.

Acne:

1. Grate a carrot, squeeze out a teaspoonful of fresh saffron-colored juice and then wipe over the blemished areas. Rinse off after a half an hour.

2. Mix a light dab of either sandalwood or turmeric powder with a little water. Dab on blemishes to clear them up.

3. Use buttermilk or watered-down yogurt as a daily face wash. Rinse with cold water.

Hair Conditioning:
1. Massage coconut oil into the scalp daily.
2. Mix a handful of hibiscus, marigold, basil and mint leaves and rose petals. Use as many ingredients as possible.

3. Grind in a blender with a little water until it forms a paste.

4. Apply directly to the scalp and hair. Leave on for at least an hour. Rinse well.

Coconut contains lauric acid, a saturated fatty acid, which binds to proteins in the hair shaft. It can improve dandruff and dry, damaged or split ends. It also improves circulation and increases hair growth.

Prana is believed to be a living life force or energy that flows through a network of fine subtle channels called nadis. It is also believed to flow through all living things including trees, water, plants and the earth. Indian women take walks in nature called a "prana walk" to absorb that surrounding energy and channel it into their bodies. This is thought to reduce stress and improve physical and mental well-being.

Native American Women's Secrets

Jojoba Oil is actually a wax ester that is similar to human skin oil.

Use as a bath oil.
Apply to hair as a conditioner to de-frizz.

Sandalwood cools and soothes the skin.

#1

1. Mix 5 tablespoons of coconut oil with 2 teaspoons of almond oil.

2. Add 4 teaspoons of sandalwood powder.
3. Apply the mixture to any area of overexposed to the sun.

4. This oil will keep your skin complexion even.

Sandalwood Oil/Powder

- Sandalwood oil can be used alone or mixed with your favorite oil.

- Can be used for a massage, conditioner or moisturizer.

Acne treatments:

#1

1. Mix 1 tsp. of sandalwood powder with 1 teaspoon of turmeric.

2. Add one tsp. of water and stir to make a paste.
3. Add a small piece of camphor for a cooling effect.
4. Apply to pimples before bedtime.

#2

1. Mix 2 tsp. of sandalwood and rosewater to make a thin paste
2. Spread it evenly on your face.

3. Leave it on for 20 to 30 minutes.
4. Rinse well.

Native American women have a long, culturally embraced history of spirituality that includes a reverence for animal life, the environment, and each other. Their beliefs were embedded in how they lived each day. How much better women could get along and successfully progress if they could embrace similar beliefs.

Modern Natural Beauty Secrets

Natural Moisturizers:

Silky Smooth Skin

1. Mix one cup of sea salt with half a cup of peppermint tea.

2. Form into a paste.
3. Can be used as a shower gel or body scrub.
4. Rinse well in bath or shower.

Plums for Beautifying Legs

Plums can reduce spider veins. They have vitamin K that helps produce thrombin, a blood-clotting protein that thickens the blood. This thicker blood is rerouted to larger, healthier blood vessels. The damaged vessels that form spider veins then shrink.

Leg beautifying sorbet

Puree in a blender:

- 12 plums (pitted, peeled and sliced)
- 1 cup of orange juice
- 3 tbs. sugar
- 1 tbs. orange zest

1. Pour into loaf pan.
2. Freeze at least 4 hours.
3. Process 30 minutes before serving.
4. Freeze until ready to eat.

Sun Proof Skin

Plums provide protection and can reverse the damage from the sun's rays. They contain vitamin A, an antioxidant that speeds up the regeneration of surface skin cells. A weekly plum facial can keep your complexion looking young and fresh.

Plum Facial Mask

In a food processor:

1. Blend 2 pitted, peeled plums and 1 egg white until smooth.
2. Gently apply mixture to face with fingertips.
3. Leave on 15 to 20 minutes.
4. Rinse skin thoroughly with cool water.

Hair

Highlight dark hair with half a cup of cranberry juice and half a cup of seltzer. Use as a final rinse after shampooing.

Sesame Coconut Hair Mask

(Restores silkiness and shine to chemically treated hair)

Combine these ingredients and mix well.

- 2 tbs. light sesame oil
- Unsweetened coconut milk
- Honey
- Avocado
- 2 eggs

1. Massage into hair after shampooing.
2. Leave on for 15-25 minutes.
3. Rinse well.

Rosemary Scalp Massage

Rosemary naturally improves circulation to the scalp and improves healthier hair growth.

Mix together:

- 10 drops of rosemary oil (available at health food stores)

- ½ cup plain full-fat yogurt
- 3 tbs. olive oil

1. Massage into dry hair.
2. Rinse well and shampoo.

Coconut Deep Conditioning Treatment

1. Microwave ¼ cup unsweetened coconut milk for 45 seconds.

2. Apply to hair.
3. Concentrate on ends.
4. Let sit 10-15 minutes.
5. Rinse well.

Shampoo and condition as usual.

Olive Oil and Lavender Scalp Treatment:(Olive oil makes hair soft and the lavender controls grease)

Mix together:

- ¼ cup olive oil
- 10 drops of lavender essential oil

1. Microwave ingredients for 45 seconds.
2. Massage into hair and scalp after shampooing.
3. Leave on for 15 minutes.
4. Rinse well.
5. Re-shampoo and condition.

Foot Massage

Try before bedtime, for at least a week.

1. Soak your feet in lukewarm water mixed with ½ cup sea salt and a tablespoon of bath gel.
2. Massage them with a mix of equal parts oil and sea salt.
3. You can use olive oil or aromatherapy oils like eucalyptus, rosemary or lavender.

4. Rinse and dry feet.
5. Coat feet with foot cream or Vaseline.
6. Wear socks to seal in softening moisture while you sleep.

Fruit Acid Restores Skin's Radiance

Cranberries contain ellagic acid, a fruit acid that dissolves toxins, dirt and germs, clearing pores and allowing more oxygen to be absorbed.

To lighten up your face scrub:

1. Puree ½ cup cranberries and 1 sliced tangerine.
2. Combine fruit mixture with ½ cup olive oil, 1 cup raw sugar, and ½ cup raw honey.

3. Stir until blended.
4. Cleanse face with scrub.
5. Rinse with tepid water.

Can store in refrigerator for up to one week.

Skin Toning Grapefruit Massage

Grapefruit holds the key to a trim belly, butt and thighs. When grapefruit oil is massaged into the skin, a compound called D-limonene stimulates the lymphatic system to flush excess fluid and toxins from bodily tissues for effortless slimming.

1. Mix 15 drops grapefruit essential oil, 1 tsp. olive oil, and ½ cup Aloe Vera gel.
2. Massage into problem area.

Can seal and store at room temperature for 1 week.

SPECIAL FACIAL SCRUBS

Azuki Bean Scrub

This scrub is an idea from Japan that is incredibly simple and has been used for hundreds of years on all skin types. To make this scrub, you will need some small dried red azuki beans, available from health food stores. Simply measure a scant cup of beans into a coffee grinder and process to a smooth powder, then store in a screw top jar. For a scrub, place 2 tablespoons of this powder in a small dish and mix it with enough water to make a smooth paste. Scrub this mixture gently over your face with small circular movements, avoiding the inner eye area. Rinse off with warm water and pat the skin dry. Your face will feel incredibly soft.

Oatmeal and Almond Scrub

This is an extremely gentle scrub that is good for all skin types, including sensitive skin. The oatmeal is cleansing and the almonds gently nourishing.

In a small dish mix together:

- 1 tbsp. of ground almonds
- 1 tbsp. of fine oatmeal

1. Add enough water to make a smooth paste.
2. Apply to the skin with small circular movements, avoiding the inner eye area.//
3. Rinse off with warm water and pat dry.

Sesame and Honey Cream

This rich liquid is marvelous for conditioning normal, mature and combination skin.

In a small dish mix together:

- 2 tablespoons of sesame oil
- 1 tbsp. of light cream
- 1 tbsp. of runny honey

1. Whisk together thoroughly, pour into a screw top jar and refrigerate.
2. The amount is enough for about four applications and will keep for up to 1 week.

Avocado and Lemon Soother

This paste is very simple.

1. Mash the pulp of half an avocado to a fine paste.
2. Add 1 teaspoon of fresh lemon juice.

This is excellent for normal and combination skin. The lemon juice lightly tones the skin and the avocado nourishes it.

These beauty secrets do wonders for our outward appearances but must be an adjunct to eating healthy, reducing stress, exercising and getting the necessary amount of sleep. Also reduce or eliminate alcohol intake, especially harsh liquors and definitely quit smoking or any illicit drug use.

Should you choose to be diligent with the above natural beauty regimes, take pride in your newfound attractiveness. However, just like the ancient goddesses, their beauty was complimented with inner strengths. It is the combination that leads to successes and conquests. Thus the lesson to be learned is: just don't work on outward beauty but also improve the essence of your inner self, which is where true beauty lies. Otherwise you will just be an empty shell, like the ones we find discarded on sandy shores.

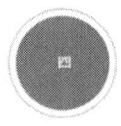

Why can I not get fit?
Lying in my bed
Downloading Netflix
Or texting friends instead

There's too much pressure
Sweating at the gym
After I just fixed my hair
It's all messed up again

I would not be concerned
But when I stepped upon the scale
It said, "Could you please get off"
"I'm unable to exhale"

CHAPTER FOUR
Not in the Gym Exercises

None of us really likes to exercise, so how can we sneak some in? Would you believe that you can begin while still in bed? As soon as you awake, open your eyes, before you roll out of bed, then shut them tightly for 3-5 seconds. Repeat these opening and closing eye movements 5X's. Slowly roll your eyes clockwise, then counter-clockwise. Stop for a second and then blink. Repeat 3X. Rub your hands together for a few seconds until they feel warm. Cup your hands over your eyes gently for a few minutes and take some relaxing breathes. These simple movements, while you're still cozy in bed improve eye health and reduce eyestrain.

Now, before you're fully out of bed, perform a few arm stretches. Sit on the side of the bed. Stretch your arms up as far as you can, hold for 5 seconds and then return them to your side. Repeat 10X for a good start. Then with arms outstretched in front of you, twist slowly to the right and then to the left. Repeat 5X.

Now you are ready to get up, a little more relaxed and taking those few minutes to realize your importance. But we're not finished. If you have stairs, go up and down them or walk up and down a hallway once or twice. That will get you moving. Do some squats while brushing your teeth, up and down, 10X should do, plus you get in that 2 minutes dentists recommend brushing your teeth. But don't floss simultaneously, you'll get directionally confused. Now relax a minute and have a nutritious breakfast. Read something inspirational to compliment your meal, it only needs to be one or two lines. Time to get back to exercising. Take exaggerated steps as you walk to your car; just ignore the neighbor's stares. Get a few neck stretches in before you start the ignition. Sit up straight and look forward. Slowly and gently bend your head forward and down, trying to touch your chin to your chest. Only go down as far as you are comfortable. Then bring your head back up to its starting position. Repeat 3X. Gently bend your head backwards and look towards the sky until you feel a slight stretch. Again return your head to the starting position. Repeat this exercise 3X. Now you are ready to start the engine (you've already started your own!) and your day. Just make sure you're not late for work, your boss will not believe this excuse.

Now, instead of trying to get the best parking spot, as close to your destination, try to park a few blocks from your destination and walk. Use stairs instead of the elevator. Also try to suck in your stomach and hold it for 20 seconds, and then push your stomach out. Repeat 10X and do that several times during the day. This simple muscle exercise will help trim your waist. You may soon be surprised at the results, especially if you're eating healthy.

Now that you've started to exercise, keep it going. The hardest part is always taking that first step.

*Of course you should always check with your health provider before starting any exercise routine. Also, any exercises that make you feel uncomfortable should be stopped immediately and seek medical assistance if needed.

Mid-Day Blues

No time to nap, mid-morning drag but still need to get moving. Mind willing but body on strike...you need instant energizers. Get "Red Bulled" naturally.

Start with breathing, a necessity of life.

Are you a chest or abdominal (diaphragmatic) breather?

Close your eyes and concentrate. Put your left palm on your chest and your right palm on your stomach. Then take a slow deep breathe. If your left hand rises more than your right hand you know you are breathing with your chest. This is how over 80% of the population breathes. However, with chest breathing, there are more breaths taken per minute but lung capacity is reduced and less oxygen exchanged.

Abdominal breathing: Sit quietly. Place your hand on your abdomen. Inhale slowly and let your abdomen expand. Hold for 1-2 seconds. Then slowly exhale allowing your abdomen to fall. Practice these 5 minutes each day and slowly work up to 20 minutes.

With abdominal breathing, the abdomen not the chest expands. This is a more natural type of breathing and actually how babies breathe. This "abdominal or diaphragmatic breathing" is also used for relaxation exercises, and a few are listed below.

Ready...Set...Blow

Bellows Breath: Sit with your back straight. With your mouth closed, inhale and exhale short breaths of equal duration very rapidly though your nose for 15 seconds only. Then resume normal breathing.

Oxygen boost: Sit with your arms stretched out at shoulder level. Then bring your arms over your head and cross your wrists. Start breathing only through your nose, which forces you to take the deeper breaths. Then breathe deeply with your whole chest and stomach for 1-5 minutes. Make sure you are comfortable while performing this technique.

Stand or sit up straight. Pull your shoulders back and tuck in your chin. Focus on abdominal breathing. Breathe in through your nose, and try to consciously expand your abdomen. As you breathe in, pull air down past your chest. Count to six, hold for 2 seconds, and then breathe out for 6 seconds, making sure to exhale through your nose and keep your mouth closed. Repeat this 10X.

Breathe in for a count of four and hold for a count of sixteen. Then release for an eight count. Keep focused on inhaling and exhaling deeply and completely. Repeat 10 X

YOGA

This ancient philosophy of mind, body and spirit is thought to originate in the East and may actually predate written history. Archeologists have found stone seals from around 3000 B.C. with pictures of yoga poses. Yoga's presence is also seen in the oldest-existing text, the Rig-Veda, a composition of hymns depicting prayer, harmony and well-being, and a foundation of Buddhist teachings.

Modern yoga is based on five principles crafted by Swami Sivananda.

- Proper relaxation
- Proper exercise
- Proper breathing
- Proper diet
- Positive thinking and meditation

This results in improved mental and physical health with a broadening of one's personal perspective on life.

Let the Stretching Begin

A proper warm up is imperative before beginning any exercise routine. This allows your muscles to become pre-stretched, making the routine easier, and reducing later muscle strain or injury. A proper warm up is especially necessary for those who exercise infrequently or are just starting to exercise, because it allows the body to recover from the shock that you are actually exercising.

Warm Up Exercises:

Shoulder Stretches

1. Keep your spine straight and your neck relaxed.
2. Slowly raise your right shoulder, and then drop it down.
3. Rest for 1-2 seconds.
4. Slowly raise your left shoulder, and then drop it down.
5. Again, rest for 1-2 seconds.
6. Raise both shoulders at once, and then drop them down again.
7. Repeat 3-5X

Neck Stretches:

All movements are performed slowly.

1. Bend your head forward bringing your chin onto your chest, then back to starting position.
2. Bend to the right, and then back to the original position.
3. Bend backward, then back to the original position.
4. Bend to the left, and then back to the original position.
5. Repeat 3-5X.

Standing Pose:

Mountain Pose (Tadasana)

1. Stand up straight with both feet at hip-width.
2. Turn your heels outward a little and let your weight rest on your toes.
3. Hang your arms downwards alongside your body with the palms of your hands pointing towards your body.
4. Now let the back of your pelvis move away from your lower back. Do this by drawing in your ribs a little towards your belly.
5. Look straight ahead and find a spot to stare at. Keep fixed on that point and stand motionless but relaxed.
6. Breathe slowly, relax and concentrate.
7. Try to stand 1-3 minutes.

Seated Pose:

The Easy Pose or Sukhasana:

1. Sit on the floor or use a Yoga Mat.
2. Cross your legs, and place your feet below your knees.
3. Clasp your hands around your knees.

4. Keep your head and body straight.
   5. Try to sit 1-3 minutes.

Finishing Poses:

Corpse Pose (Savasana)

   1. Lie on your back with your arms and legs stretched out
   2. Rotate your legs gently inward and then outward. Do not lift them off the floor, and then gently let them fall out to the sides.

   3. Let your arms fall alongside your body, slightly separated from the body, with palms facing upwards.

   4. Rotate the spine by turning your head from side to side until you feel it centered.

   5. Start stretching yourself out, as though someone is pulling your head away from your feet. Keep your shoulders down and away from your neck and your legs down and away from your pelvis.

Now for those who have mastered the basic yoga postures and want to be a little more challenged, here are a few more advanced yoga poses.

What is the difference between you and a pretzel? A pretzel can do these exercises.

Modified Down-Dog Split:

   1. Start in a pushup position. Slowly lift your hips.
   2. Move into a downward facing dog. Stop. Take five breaths.

3. Raise your right heel stretching toward the ceiling. Then slowly lower your left forearm to the floor. Keep both palms flat on the floor.

Warrior 3:

1. Straighten your left arm.
2. Place your right foot between your hands.
3. As you raise your left leg, shift your weight onto your right foot. At the same time, raise your torso until it is parallel to the floor. Reach your arms forward.

Modified Half-Moon Arch:

1. Place both hands on the floor beneath your shoulders.
2. Rotate your hips to the left.
3. Raise your left arm toward the ceiling. Bend your left knee back.
4. Reach your left hand behind you to hold your foot.

Tree:

1. From half-moon arch, turn your hips and shoulders back toward the floor.
2. Use your core muscles to roll your body up to a standing position.
3. Place the sole of your left foot on your right inner thigh. Lift both arms straight up above your shoulders.

Body of Evidence

If these exercises work just give me a toe tag.

Facial Exercises

Eyes

1. Sit comfortably. Rub your hands together until they begin to feel warm. Close your eyes. Cover them lightly with your cupped palms. Do not apply pressure to your eyeballs and keep your nose uncovered. Focus on the darkness. Take slow deep breaths until you see nothing but blackness. Remove your palms from your eyes. Repeat for 3 minutes.

2. Close your eyes tightly for 3-5 seconds. Then open them for 3-5 seconds. Repeat 8 times.

3. Close your eyes. With your fingers, massage them with circular movements for 1-2 minutes. Press very lightly and make sure your hands are washed.

4. First roll your eyes clockwise, then counter-clockwise. Blink in between each time. Repeat 5 times

Chest exercises

We must develop the bust because it's better for sweaters.

These exercises are designed to strengthen the chest muscles. Because the muscles actually lie under the breast, doing these exercises make the breast firmer, not bigger.

Chest Fly

Lie face up on the mat. Bend your knees but keep your feet flat on the floor. Use a light- to medium-weight dumbbells and place in both hands. Keep your arms at a slight bend. Raise your arms straight up. Keep palms facing each other. Slowly let your arms fall out to the side and then bring them back together, returning to the starting position. Repeat 3-8X.

Ball Squeeze

Hold a medium-sized ball (something the size of a basketball) in both hands and keep it right in front of your chest. Squeeze the ball as hard as you can and hold for five counts and then release. Repeat 3-8X.

Push Ups

To strengthen your chest and shoulders:

Step 1. Walk your hands out until they are just beneath your shoulders.

Step 2. Contract your abdominal muscles. Bend at the elbows. Keep your body in a straight line from your shoulders to your knees. Lower your chin just above your fingers.

Step 3. Exhale as you press up to return to the starting position.

Repeat 10 times.

Arm Circles

To strengthen your shoulders:

Step 1. Stand with feet together
Step 2. Slightly bend at your knees. Keep your back straight
Step 3. Put your left hand on your hip. Extend your right arm directly in front of you at shoulder height.

Step 4. Move your arm in small clockwise circles while keeping the rest of your body still.

Once you've completed 10 reps, change directions. Do 10 more counter clockwise circles? Switch arms and repeat.

Leg Exercises

#1

1. Gently place an exercise ball between the wall and the curve of your lower back.

2. Stand with your feet shoulder apart, about 3-5 inches.
3. Keep your shoulders level, back straight, and bend knees about 5 to 10 inches.

4. Hold this position for 3 seconds and then stand back up to starting position.

5. Start with 5 reps, rest for 30 seconds and do another set.

#2

1. Lie back on the mat, arms by your sides and palms facing down.
2. Start by pointing your left foot, reaching out with your toes toward the ceiling, and rotate your leg slightly outward.

3. Inhale, and then trace a circle on the ceiling with your left leg.

4. Do this 5 times in a clockwise direction and repeat 5 times in a counter-clockwise direction. Switch legs and repeat. Do 5 repetitions.

#3

1. Stand behind a chair and hold the back of it.
2. Press your shoulder blades back and down.
3. Come up on the ball of your left foot, and lift your right leg.

4. Keep both hips facing forward.

5. Bring your right leg across your body, in front of your left.

6. Now, swing it back out to the right.
7. Keeping toes flexed and turned out
8. Do 10 reps.
9. Switch legs and repeat

Buttocks Exercises

#1

1. Lie face up on floor with legs extended.
2. Keep heels resting on the seat of a chair with arms by sides and palms down

3. Lift right leg straight over hip.
4. Keep foot flexed.

5. Slowly lift hips off floor until body forms a straight line from left heel to left shoulder then lower.
6. Do 20 reps
7. Switch legs; repeat.

#2

1. Stand with feet shoulder-width apart and arms by sides.

2. Squat slowly to the count of 4
3. Both knees are bent 90 degrees.
4. Both arms are straight and raised to shoulder level in front of you.

5. Repeat 10X.

#3

1. Stand on your tiptoes with feet together.

2. Stand a couple of feet behind chair with hands on the back of the chair.

3. Keeping back flat, hinge forward slightly from waist.
4. Lift bent left knee to hip level in front of you.
5. Place left foot by right knee.
6. Push back to resting position
7. Repeat 10 times.

Even with a gym membership, you don't always have time to get there. However, you usually make it home, eventually.

Remember, exercises can be done at anytime, so don't limit yourself. You can listen to music or watch TV while doing them. Make yourself comfortable. Always do a 5-10 minute warm up and cool down before and after exercising. Warm-ups could include light calisthenics, jogging, jumping jacks, or comfortable walking up and down several flights of stairs. The cooling down period, after the workout, involves less strenuous exercises with stretching, deep breathing and relaxation. The important thing is to find a way to fit it in some type of exercise program and be consistent.

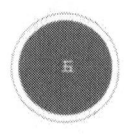

I try to look away but you call out my name
Although silently whispered, I can hear just the same
In the darkest of night and earliest day
Into my world, you still find a way

Despite my strong will I always succumb
But thoroughly enjoy the fact that you've won
So I hang my head low, despite beaten again
And stuff my face full of chocolate sin

CHAPTER FIVE
Healthy Eating

Being a little older, a little fatter and/or less healthy drives most to want to get back on the right nutritional track. However, the real key is fitting "healthy eating" into an entrenched and lifelong established habit of poor eating. It is easier to grab something on the go, super-size, justify binge eating, or eat what tastes good. To compensate, just buy clothes in a bigger size or with an elastic waistband.

Then you reach a point where you want to become serious about what you eat because it does have a significant impact on how you look, act and feel. Laden weight is burdensome when negotiating a flight of stairs, doing routine housework, or just trying to keep up with a grandchild's youth. Dieting is now mandatory if life is to be enjoyed, not just sustained. Now desperately looking for the road that allows one the advertised success to release the "slimmer me inside". But how? I cannot turn into a rabbit that nibbles on carrots and lettuce all day because God did not create me with a tail and "buck teeth". Also with today's economy, I would not do well trying to raise a litter.

The true answers lie in education, determination and balance. Learn from the myriad of foods out there what you like that is healthy. Be determined to create and follow a pathway of healthier eating. Finally, balance it with what you can afford, have reasonably available, and is satisfying.

EDUCATION

Education comes from the ability to listen before you learn.

In January 2011, the USDA Center for Nutrition Policy and Promotion (CNPP) announced its 2010 Dietary Guidelines for Americans, in an effort to improve population health. Wise-choice dietary selections were encouraged from the five food groups: vegetables, fruits, whole grains, fat-free and low-fat dairy products, and seafood. They also advised consuming less or avoiding altogether sodium, saturated and trans fats, added sugars, and refined grains.

The concept of 'MyPlate' replaced the traditional 'MyPyramid' to associate the more familiar "place setting" when planning a meal and thinking about food choices. It emphasizes how to get the maximum nutrition out of calorie choices and make smart choices from the individual food groups. Reducing total calorie consumption, staying within your calorie needs, and increasing physical activity is strongly encouraged.

These Dietary Guidelines also suggest the following to help Americans implement these changes into their everyday lives:

Enjoy your food, but eat less.
Avoid oversized portions.
Make half your plate fruits and vegetables.
Switch to fat-free or low-fat (1%) milk.

Compare sodium in foods like soup, bread, and frozen meals – and choose the foods with lower numbers.

Drink water instead of sugary drinks.

(The 2010 Dietary Guidelines are available at www.dietaryguidelines.gov.)

This information is helpful in determining what to eat, but how does it fit into an individual's lifestyle successfully?

I. How to triumph over hunger pains?

That is the downfall of most diets and implementing these healthy nutritional changes, the brain is willing but the mouth is unable to comply. Deprivation married to those tempting hunger pains will eventually defeat the most dedicated. Without a balance between hunger and satiety (feeling full), chocolate cake just looks too good.

Quick tips to fight hunger:

Do:

- Try to drink 6-8 glasses of water each day. It has no calories, stretches the stomach and activates certain receptors that make the brain think you are full.

- Drink a glass of vegetable juice before meals. You will eat less.

- Drink green tea. It is an appetite suppressant and fat burner.

- Eat foods high in fiber. This adds bulk to food without adding calories. Good sources of fiber are dried beans, bran, vegetables, and whole grains.

- Munch on an apple. They are rich in pectin, a soluble fiber that slows the digestive process, making you feel full on less food.

- Eat energy dense fruits (grapes, avocados, coconuts, dried fruits and watermelon) and energy dense vegetables (cucumbers, tomatoes, jicama, broccoli, beets, carrots or celery). They are abundant in water and lower in calories.

- Chew gum an hour in the morning. Scientists believe the chewing motion sends signals to the brain that make you feel full. You will eat fewer calories at lunch.

- Keep 100 calorie snacks around the house at all times but only have 2-3/day.

- Eat 2 small pieces of dark chocolate. It contains steric acid that helps slow digestion. Also the bitter taste decreases appetite.

Multiple scents and aromas may decrease appetite. These include vanilla, cranberries, peppermint, lemon and the essential oils fennel and patchouli.

When you eat out, have just enough to feel satisfied. Bring leftovers home for a later treat.

Don't:

- If you are really hungry, don't go out to eat, you will just overeat.

- Don't splurge on a favorite food unless you've earned it and have stayed on some type of healthy eating program for at least a week. You will just use it as an excuse to keep splurging.

- Get enough sleep. Your body increases the hormone ghrelin, which stimulates appetite and decreases the hormone leptin that helps you lose weight if you are sleep deprived. Take a nap the next day to make up if you have not been able to sleep well the previous night.

- Don't skip breakfast; you will eat more during the day to make-up. Have at least a granola bar, toast or piece of fruit.

- Don't say, "I really don't eat that much". Keep a food diary for one week and you will see how much you really eat. If you truly think your weight excess is due to a medical problem, have your doctor check for underactive thyroid problems and diabetes.

- Don't keep doing what you are doing; you will just get what you have always got. Change is good, embrace it and develop ways to eat healthier. Learn to like fruits and vegetables; there are a lot to choose from.

- Don't give into cravings. Suck on mints, chew gum or find something to keep you busy for 10 minutes. Most of those cravings are impulse driven and go away with time.

II. Improving Mental Focus

ZINC

Zinc is an important element in the body. It may enhance communication between brain cells that facilitates learning and improves memory. It has also been shown to improve eyesight, taste, smell, hair, skin and boosts the immune system. Excellent sources include beef, lamb, pork, chicken and turkey. Shellfish sources are crab, lobster, clams, salmon, oysters, herring and mussels. Almonds, apricots, peanuts, pine nuts, cashews, sunflower and pumpkin seeds are non-meat sources of zinc. Bran, multi-grain and whole grain cereals are often found fortified with zinc.

Green Tea

The brain needs a high amount of oxygen to carry out its metabolism (chemical reactions in the cell that sustain life). This can often lead to the formation of free radicals as a by-product, which are unstable molecules and can damage brain cells. Some scientists feel these free radicals may be related to the development of cancer. Green tea contains the anti-oxidants polyphenols and flavonoids, which reduces the amount of free radicals. It also reduces the amounts of beta amyloid proteins thought to be involved with the formation of brain plaques, implicated in nerve damage and memory loss.

Additional benefits of green tea may include: lowering cholesterol, better heart health, boosts the immune system, cancer prevention, and assists with weight loss.

GABA (gamma amino butyric acid).

GABA is found in nerve tissues, especially in the brain and suppresses nerve activity. Supplemented in the diet, it is thought to balance out mood swings, reduce anxiety, and help keep your composure. Excellent food sources are eggs, yogurt, and fish - especially salmon.

Non-Heme Iron

Heme is an iron-containing substance. It combines with the protein "globin" to form hemoglobin, found in the red blood cells. These cells are important for carrying oxygen the body needs to nourish other cells and provide energy. Heme may also be important in maximizing brain activity.

Heme-iron is the iron that comes from meats like beef and chicken, while non-heme iron is obtained from plants. Good vegetarian sources include soybeans, lentils, lima beans, black-eyed peas, and black/pinto beans. Dark green leafy vegetables like spinach, turnip greens, and swiss chard contain high amounts of iron. Try to incorporate broccoli, bok choy, tofu, and quinoa into your meals - they are not only rich in flavor, but also in nutrients. Vitamin C increases the body's ability to absorb non-heme iron, and is found in citrus fruits: oranges, lemons, limes, and grapefruits.

Both nutrients are found in these tasty treats. Try red and yellow bell peppers dipped in hummus, stir-fried and served over iron-enriched rice or added to your favorite chicken salad. Try chutney toppings over meats that include lemons or oranges.

Blueberry

These berries contain antioxidants called anthocyanin. They may speed up communication between brain cells that improve memory, decision making and reasoning skills. They may help lower cholesterol, strengthen blood vessels, improve eye health, and have some anticancer benefits.

III. POWER PRODUCE

Celery is a vegetable that is rich in vitamins and minerals. Its leaves contain vitamin A and stems vitamins B1, B2, B6 and C. Minerals include potassium, folic acid, calcium, magnesium, iron, phosphorus, sodium and plenty essential amino acids. Some research shows it may lower blood pressure and fight cancer. The fiber in celery helps regulate bowel movements. It's tasteless, but good for strengthening a recipe. Add it to your favorite soups or include in potato, chicken or tuna salads, and dressing for turkeys.

Potato: Don't fry it or load the baked version with fat and salt heavy calories, and you'll find that the potato can be quite nutritional. Its cholesterol lowering fiber also regulates digestion. It contains magnesium which improves bone health, immune boosting Vitamin C, and kukoamine that lowers blood pressure. In addition, the spud contains Vitamin B, folate and the minerals potassium, copper and iron. The skin contains flavanoids that protect the heart. It lowers LDL (the bad cholesterol☐) which helps keep the arteries unclogged and Vitamin B6 which reduces the level of a molecule called homocysteine, thought to cause to heart attacks and strokes.

Parsley: This festive herb is more than just a garnish for special recipes. It is rich in antioxidants, especially apigenin, which may help reduce the risk of breast, colon, and skin cancers. Parsley is rich in the vitamins A and C, and K and a good source of iron and folate. It is rich in volatile oils that give off an astringent flavor that inhibits the activity elements harmful to the body.

Watermelon: This sweet, tasty fruit that is low-fat, nutritionally dense and loaded with water, which is life essential. They are excellent sources of vitamin A, important in eye health, and vitamin C that boosts immunity and keeps gums and teeth healthy. Its vitamin B6 helps brain function.

Avoid Energy drain

Have you ever wondered why you feel sleepy after lunch? There is a natural dip in the body's blood sugar between 3p.m. and 5p.m., just the time when most of us are struggling at work in those last few hours of the day. Also there is a natural drop in your core temperature about eight hours after you get up in the morning

To combat this downshift, enjoy foods rich in Vitamin B (like chicken, tuna or sliced avocado) for lunch. B-complex vitamins slow digestion, keep blood sugar steady and maximize the absorption of other nutrients. Pumpkin and sunflower seeds are also rich in vitamin - a quick snack that gives you a boost of energy. Keep well hydrated and drink plenty of water.

The aroma of spice and citrus combats tiredness. Cinnamon oils increase energizing blood flow to the brain and muscles. Lime oil improves focus. Blend with basil to further stimulate the brain and body. Ginger scents invigorate nerves and combat tiredness. Try combining with grapefruit to synergize the effects. Place a few drops of these essential oils in a scented warmer and add not just spice but energy to your office.

Add Quality Oils to your Diet

(use in small amounts as they can be high in calories)

Olive Oil

Olive oil is made from pressed ripe olives and the first cold pressing (extra virgin) yields the best quality. They contain monounsaturated fatty acids that lower total cholesterol and low-density lipoprotein (LDL) cholesterol levels. They may also affect insulin levels and improve blood sugar control. These lubricating oils are good for the hair, face and skin. Store olive oil at room-temperature in a dark, cupboard and use within 6 months of opening.

Sunflower-Seed Oil

Many people are unaware that sunflowers can produce oil and are rich in vitamins A, D, and antioxidants and phytochemicals, including vitamin E, betaine, phenolic acid, choline, arginine and lignans various minerals. Antioxidants fight free radicals and prevent cell damage.

Sesame Oil

This oil is a favorite in Chinese, Middle Eastern, and Indian cooking. Rich in vitamin E, calcium, magnesium and phosphorus, it is also used extensively for hair and skin therapies. Use approximately 2 tablespoons of these excellent oils each day in cooking and salads daily. The body can easily process the fat in these oils; it also helps with digestion.

Essential Minerals

Calcium

- Calcium is needed for many functions of the body.
- It promotes the growth and formation of the bones and teeth

- It maintains the heart and muscles
- Its presence in the tissue helps to speed up the healing process

- It helps nutrients pass through cell walls
- It helps the body use minerals such as iron to form blood cells

When calcium levels are low, the body's reaction can be diverse. Low calcium levels can cause dehydration of the skin, or premenstrual syndrome. Complications with osteoporosis and bone and teeth deficiencies have been associated with poor calcium levels.

Fortunately, calcium is contained in many foods across the various food groups. Foods to enjoy that will also provide calcium include: oily fish, milk, cheese, eggs, soybeans (used to make tofu), chickpeas and corn.

Many green vegetables also contain calcium including: spinach, arugula, broccoli, kale, mustard and collard greens, watercress, and salad onions.

Young dandelion leaves found in spring, taste delicious in salads. Calcium is also found in seaweed, which is a common ingredient in Japanese dishes. Seaweed is used in the preparation of sushi. Almonds and sunflower seeds, as we have already seen are also good sources of calcium.

WATER

Water filters the kidneys. The kidneys clean the body of the toxins we accumulate on a daily basis.

Water is vital to the human body, but is also is beneficial to the appearance of the skin and face. The Department of Health recommends drinking 6-8 large glasses (about 8 ½ cups) of water daily. Pure spring water is suggested. It may sound like a lot, but this is an easy target to attain.

For the spring water connoisseur, a number of varieties have appeared on the market. When it comes to these "gourmet" waters, French mineral waters are considered to be some of the finest waters in the world. French standards for analysis, purity and mineral content are extremely well established. Water from the mountain region of the Auvergne is considered to be particularly pure. In France, many doctors advise their patients to drink mineral water to help conditions such as water retention or urinary problems.

FOODS TO EAT AND LOOSE WEIGHT

Chili Powder

Capsicum, (kap-si-kem) which is found in chili peppers work as an appetite suppressant. A recent study from the Netherlands found that when people drank tomato juice spiked with hot pepper over a two -day period, they consumed up to 16 percent fewer calories over the next two days. They also felt more satisfied than when they consumed a blander version of the same juice. Capsicum has been proven to be an effective anti-inflammatory, a potent antioxidant and a promising cancer fighter. Scientist at the University of California, Los Angeles, found that giving mice this compound caused prostate cancer cells to self - destruct.

Spice Up Your Diet: Sprinkle chili powder on macaroni and cheese or corn on the cob, or tomato soup. Add hot sauce to eggs and omelets.

Try: spicy hummus instead of: Creamy dressing

Slim Down Recipe: Mix ½ teaspoon of chili powder into a small tub of commercially prepared hummus. Scoop out a two-tablespoon serving and bring on the veggies.

- You save: 100 calories, 13 fat grams

Cinnamon

Antioxidant and antibacterial properties

A study conducted at the University of Illinois at Chicago, suggested that a cinnamon flavored gum might fight bad breath. The U.S. Department of Agriculture (USDA) researchers stated that cinnamon might also aid in glucose control. Having as little as ½ teaspoon of cinnamon daily can improve blood glucose levels and lower cholesterol, particularly in people with type- 2 diabetes.

Spice Up Your Diet: Sprinkle cinnamon on squash or sweet potatoes, or add a little to coffee grounds before you brew.

Try: Blueberry hot cereal instead of: Instant oatmeal

Slim Down Recipe: Combine ½ cup rolled oats to 1 cup of water. Cook. Stir in ½ cup of frozen blueberries and ½ teaspoon of cinnamon.

- You save: 100 calories

Note: Keep A Lid On It Dried herbs and spices last only nine months to a year. Write the date of purchase on the lids with a marker or keep a list inside a kitchen cabinet. When a color or scent fades, it's time to replace them.

Garlic:

Garlic has earned fame as a powerful health aid. It is rich in organo-sulfur compounds, with high levels of antioxidant activity. Garlic releases the antibiotic allicin when chopped or crushed. British researchers recently reinforced the validity of the benefits of garlic, by reviewing all clinical trials published on garlic's effect on cardiovascular disease since 1993. They concluded that despite mixed findings, science does suggest that garlic reduces cholesterol and thins the blood. It also helps lower the risk of heart disease and stroke, while increasing the levels of disease fighting antioxidants in the body.

The benefits of garlic continue to inspire researchers to look for additional uses for medicinal purposes. A study from Anna Malai University in India suggests that garlic may help fight cancer, and is especially powerful when combined with the chemicals in tomatoes.

Spice Up Your Diet: Sprinkle chopped or crushed garlic on pizza; add it to salsas, sauces and marinades; or roast whole cloves and spread on a crusty loaf of bread instead of butter

Try: tomato salad instead of: potato salad

Slim Down Recipe: Chop and seed six fresh tomatoes (approximately 2 pounds), mix with 1 tablespoon olive oil, two minced cloves of garlic and red wine vinegar to taste (makes approximately four 1-cup servings).

- You save: 292 calories, 17 fat grams

Rosemary

This "piney" flavored herb boasts high levels of antioxidants, as it contains two powerful free radical eliminators, carnosol and rosmarinic acid. Research shows that rosemary may help fight cancers of the breast, lung and skin. The antioxidant activity in rosemary can reduce the production of heterocyclic amines, carcinogens that form when meats are cooked at extremely high temperatures (like on the grill). The benefits of using rosemary acts as a food safety feature when grilling food.

Spice Up Your Diet: Mix it in an aromatic marinade for grilled chicken; spruce up stuffing with a couple of teaspoons or use fresh sprigs as skewers for shish kebabs on the grill (just be sure to soak them in water first so they don't catch fire).

Try: Rosemary spiced red potatoes instead of: Potato chips and dip

Slim Down Recipe: Stir four medium size red potatoes into six wedges each. Toss with 2 teaspoons olive oil, 1 teaspoon crushed dried rosemary and a pinch of salt. Bake at 450 $°$, stirring occasionally, until the potatoes are tender and the edges are crisp (makes four servings: six wedges each).

- You save: 6 calories, 13 fat grams

Note: Storage Hints

Heat and ultraviolet light break down the chemicals in dried herbs and spices, so keep them in a cool, dark drawer or cabinet rather than in a rack that sits on top of the counter near the stove.

Curry Powder

Turmeric, an ingredient in curry powder, contains curcumin. This phytochemical helps thwart cancer by "switching off" proteins that cause cells to multiply and by inducing cancer cells to self-destruct. The spice my also reduce risk of Alzheimer, psoriasis and arthritis.

Spice Up Your Diet: Add it to bean based soups, stir into plain yogurt for an exotic dip or sprinkle on pineapple slices and grill for a tasty side dish.

Try: Curry Tuna Crunch instead of: Tuna Salad

Slim Down Recipe: Mix 1 tablespoon low fat mayo with 1 tablespoon plain low fat yogurt, one 6 ounce can of water packed chunk light tuna (drained), ½ to ½ teaspoon of curry powder, 1 tablespoon chopped walnuts, ¼ tart apples (chopped) and 1 tablespoon chopped celery.

- You save: 181 calories, 14 fat grams

Oregano

This aromatic herb, most often associated with Italian and Greek cuisines, contain quercertin and rosemarinic acids, both strong antioxidants. Scientists at the USDA have shown that 1 tablespoon of fresh oregano offers as much antioxidant activity as a medium sized apple. In fact, gram for gram, oregano packs the biggest antioxidant punch of any culinary herb. Although experts aren't sure whether dried oregano has the same level as fresh, it won't hurt to add either to your diet – especially since other research suggests that it may protect against breast, ovarian and endometrial cancers.

Spice Up Your Diet: Sprinkle fresh or dried oregano on pizza, add to oven-roasted veggies or mix it into low fat plain yogurt with garlic and lemon juice for a Greek inspired grilled sandwich spread.

Try: Mediterranean Eggs instead of: A Cheddar Omelet

Slim Down Recipe: Whisk together one whole egg and two egg whites and pour into a medium skillet coated with nonfat cooking spray. When partially set, sprinkle with ½ ounce of feta cheese, one small-diced plum tomato and ¼ to ½ teaspoon dried oregano.

- You save: 122 calories, 13 fat grams

Cumin

A main player in Indian, Mexican, Caribbean and North African cuisines, this antioxidant rich spice has been shown to lower blood glucose levels. It may also protect against stomach ulcers and gastric cancer by killing the H. pylori bacteria.

Spice UP Your Diet: Add cumin to enchiladas and tacos, rub it on meats, or sprinkle it on scrambled eggs.

Try: Tex Mex Black Beans instead of: Baked Beans

Slim Down Recipe: Mix together one 16 ounce can of black beans; one 15 ounce can of corn, both drained and rinsed; ½ cup of jarred "chunky" salsa; 1 to 2 teaspoons ground cumin; the juice of one lime; 1 tablespoons ground cumin; the juice of one lime; 1 tablespoon olive oil; and salt and pepper to taste (makes four servings, just under 1 cup each).

- You save: 145 calories, 8 fat grams

When you double a recipe that uses bold herbs and spices like ginger, curry and cumin), use only one and a half times the original amount. Otherwise, the taste might be too pungent.

Clearly eating healthy starts with knowing what to eat but also enjoying what you eat. There is such a variety to choose from and look it not as a diet but changing eating habits that incorporate easily into your lifestyle. You can still have occasional "splurges" and foods you enjoy, but balance with healthier eating and exercise. Most important, simplify, start slow, and progress at your own pace to be successful.

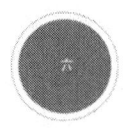

To Dr. X

It's a good thing my brain has no color
For you to label it the other
Thank God I will always be free
Of the chains you try to put on me

My dreams started long ago
Caring allowed my feelings to grow
For people I wanted to reach out
And cure the ills where there was doubt

I studied hard and made the grade
My dues I certainly did pay
Sometimes I didn't know where to begin
I kept the candle burning at both ends

The real difficulty concerned my peers
Was it my black skin that made them sneer
Did they think that cornrows had tightened my brain?
And cause me to think I was insane

What about the woman who fell on the floor
Shouting I can't take it no more
Sitting in an emergency room for hours
Who allowed you to have such power

Don't snicker and sneer cause they're Medicaid
Help them, that's why you were trained
Not to appease a hospital chief
Or bow to the point you have no belief

So the next time your telephone rings
Concerning a patient that needs to be seen

Don't succumb and become a person who pouts
Let in the sun and the good will come out

CHAPTER SIX
Dietary Changes for Common Health Problems

These dietary suggestions are for informational purposes only and should not be used as exclusive treatments for any medical disorders. Do not stop taking your prescription medications and always consult your health care provider before making any changes in your diet or medications.

The poems in this chapter were written to compel exposure to the reality of healthcare as it exists today, which is not good. Not to take away from the many truly dedicated physicians, administrators, health care workers and supportive staff, that have given their best time and effort in providing quality care, but on the larger scale, their voices are muted. Lost is medical excellence, in the escalating administrative strangulations that replace quality for quantity and smiles for sound judgments. Patient satisfaction surveys ridered to financial reimbursements have a greater importance than positive patient outcomes, which can only come from experienced professionally –made decisions.

But also the medical professional is not unscathed. Deprived of advancements based on medical performance, we have instead used at least five of the seven deadly sins, greed, sloth, lust, envy and gluttony, to catapult our standing in an insalubrious medical environment. We know patients are not receiving the care they deserve from us. However, some of us find that part easy to not recognize or there would have been more of a vocal force from our medical community. Yes, we remain inundated with escalating malpractice, frivolous lawsuits, hospital political anarchy, unappreciated work, but to allow this to let us loose our voice....unacceptable.

Order sets, the peripheral brain that predetermines what test a health care provider should order, has taken away from the needed critical thinking required to make sound medical judgments. As a result, an unnecessary myriad of test are performed, hoping that some positive result will make the diagnosis, we are no longer medically trained to make.

Medicine is not a business, it is an art of caring. Although much time, study and stamina are pre-requisites, their purpose is only to strengthen the art, not replace it. That doesn't mean the business side of medicine is not important, but belongs in the conducting of good solid business practices, not in making medical decisions, unqualified to make.

Unless dismantled, and appropriately rebuilt, the future of medicine will only result in descending us further down the health hill until the bottom is reached. The only benefit is that we will be easier to bury.

With rising health care cost and limited access to health care, one is forced to take an interest in one's own personal health, especially in an obesity-riddled society, plagued with the insurgence of complex medical problems like diabetes, hypertension and heart disease. Choices made now affect not only quality, but the duration of one's life as well. Unfortunately, there is no magic pill to erase the long-standing and deleterious effects of smoking, excess drinking, personalized stresses, depression driven binges, inexcusable illicit drug use or fat-laden diets. However, it is never too late, even if you have already been diagnosed with an ailment, to make a serious change towards a better lifestyle. However, it does not come without paying a toll. Serious commitment, behavioral medications, and a sincere willingness are prerequisites, and allegiance is mandatory.

Listed below are some common health disorders. With a few simple dietary changes, reasonable exercise, and an improved mental outlook, many can reduce medication needs, disease progression and improve outcomes.

Heart Disease

Women with heart disease may have different symptoms than their male counterparts. Instead of the well-associated crushing "chest pains" often indicative of heart ailments, women complain of less severe pain, pressure or discomfort in the chest. Other symptoms include shortness of breath, nausea or vomiting, sweating, dizziness, fatigue, neck, shoulder, upper back or abdominal discomfort

FACTS

- 42 million American women live with cardiovascular disease.

- One out of every two women or about 500,000 each year may lose their life to heart disease.

- More than 8 million women have a history of heart attack and/or angina.

- Heart disease is the number one killer of women and in the United States.

Lloyd-Jones D, Adams R, Brown T.Et al. Heart Disease and Stroke Statistics 2010 Update: A Report from the American Heart Association Statistics Committee and Stroke Statistics Subcommittee. Circulation. 2010; 121:e1-e170.

What more needs to be said?

Heart disease is a problem most of us or someone we care about, our mother, wife, sister, aunt, grandmother, cousin, partner or close friend either face, or will face, but one that can be conquered. Understanding heart disease is a good start, and doing something about it is a better one.

Heart disease affects the heart and/or the blood vessels that nourish and provide oxygen. High cholesterol, high blood pressure, smoking, alcohol, stress, obesity, and women who suffer complications during pregnancy, like preeclampsia and gestational diabetes are at greater risk. Unfortunately, because women dismiss warning symptoms as less serious conditions, they often show up to the emergency room with significant heart damage already established.

Coronary artery disease (CAD) is the most common type of heart disease. It comes from hard plaque deposits, comprised mostly of fat, cholesterol and calcium that build up on the inner walls of major blood vessels. Over time, this narrows their openings, reducing the flow of oxygen-rich blood. Lurking as a silent killer, this process can progress slowly over time and eventually lead to chest pain, damage to the heart muscle, and eventually heart disease or a heart attack. Other vital organs, like the brain and kidneys, can also become damaged.

Coronary microvascular disease (MVD) occurs when the smaller blood vessels that nourish the heart are affected by a similar process. Their tiny walls are damaged, and a smaller area is affected. This type of heart disease is more common in women and instead of the "crushing" chest pain seen in CAD, their symptoms are more subtle and often ignored.

A heart-healthy diet can be beneficial and assist in reducing this artery-clogging process for both CAD and MVD.

DIET:

"Keep your diet low in saturated fat, cholesterol and salt. Drink lots of water, exercise, maintain normal weight, reduce stress, and avoid smoking, drugs and alcohol."

Make sure you choose the good fats

Good fats are needed in the diet, so you should know which ones are healthier. Good fats help absorb important fat-soluble vitamins (A, D, E and K), contribute to the body's energy needs, play a role in proper growth, support metabolism, and give your skin a healthy glow. Choose monosaturated and polyunsaturated fats, and reduce or avoid saturated and transfats.

Increasing monosaturated and polyunsaturated oils reduce saturated fat intake. These include olive (extra virgin), canola, peanut, sunflower, safflower, sesame, corn, grapeseed, cottonseed and soybean oil. Omega-3 fatty acids are an "essential" fatty acid, which means they cannot be manufactured by our body. In order to function properly, our body needs to get these from our diet. Other good sources are olives, nuts, soy, flaxseed, walnuts, peanut butter and avocados. Fish, like salmon, mackerel, herring, cod, tuna and halibut, area good source of omega-3 fatty acids. However, be cautious and conscious of your fish intake, as the FDA recommends, "...that no more than 12 ounces of low mercury fish should be consumed weekly," for children and women who are, or are trying, to get pregnant."Highest Level Mercury" fish should be avoided and "High Level Mercury" fish should be kept to only three 6-oz servings per month. Examples of both are listed below.

Highest Level Mercury

- Marlin
- Orange roughly
- Tilefish

- Swordfish
- Shark
- Mackerel (King)
- Tuna (Bigeye, Ahi)

High Level Mercury

- Sea Bass (Chilean)
- Bluefish
- Grouper
- Mackerel (Spanish, Gulf)
- Tuna (Canned, White albacore)
- Tuna (Yellow fin)

American Pregnancy Association: Promoting Pregnancy Wellness,http://americanpregnancy.org/pregnancyhealth/fish mercury.htm (January 201.

Stay away from saturated fats, found in red meats, whole-milk dairy products, cheese, sour cream, ice cream, and butter. Cocoa butter, palm oil, coconut oil and coconut milk are other sources and some may be hidden ingredients in chocolate, cookies, cakes, non-dairy whipped toppings and coffee creamers.

Avoid transfats. They are used to extend the shelf life of processed foods. Typically, trans fat products include cookies, cakes, fries, donuts, "hydrogenated oil" or "partially hydrogenated oil," processed meats (meat preserved by smoking, curing or salting) like bacon and sausage, ham, pastrami, hot dogs and luncheon meats.

Lower LDL cholesterol (the "bad" cholesterol) and raise HDL (the "good" cholesterol).

LDL is an abbreviation forlow-density lipoprotein. It is considered the "bad" cholesterol because it can build up in the walls of blood vessels, causing them to narrow, and reduce needed and nourishing blood flow to vital body cells. HDL is an abbreviation for high-density lipoprotein. This type of cholesterol, found in the bloodstream, removes harmful "LDL" cholesterol. HDL cholesterol also transports it to the liver where it is reused and recycled. It is very important to keep HDL cholesterol levels greater than 60 milligrams per deciliter and LDL cholesterol levels less than 100 milligrams per deciliter.

Eat fresh fruits and vegetables and eliminate those fried, breaded, and frozen foods, especially those frozen foods in heavy syrup, cream sauces or with added sugars. Choose fruits and vegetables high in antioxidants, folate, fiber and potassium. These include avocados, papayas, strawberries, oranges, broccoli, bell peppers, kale, mustard greens, raspberries and carrots.

Salt consumption should be reduced to, or less than, 2000 milligrams (mg) a day and adequate potassium intake is, 700 milligrams (mg) each day. Avoid adding salt; instead season with fresh herbs such as: basil, tarragon, turmeric, chives, oregano, rosemary, sage, thyme and mint. Limit the intake of salty foods, bouillon cubes, powdered broths, soups, gravies, soy sauce, salami, bacon, cured meats, pretzels and potato chips. Look for those products using sea salt instead of regular salt. Table salt is highly refined which removes magnesium and trace minerals. In addition, various additives like aluminum compounds are added. Because .the natural iodine is destroyed during the refining process, so it is necessary to add potassium iodide.

Sea salt is sun dried, not refined. It also contains small amounts of sea life, which provides natural iodine and additional minerals. The flavor is stronger, so less salt is needed.

Good sources of potassium are orange juice, bananas, cantaloupe, tomatoes, avocados, potatoes and lima beans.

Always check food labels to make sure you know exactly what you are eating.

Limit sugar, those tempting simple carbohydrates found in sweets, sweets, sweets (cake, cookies, pies, pastries, sodas). Learn portion sizes; get a scale and some measuring cups if needed. Limit pasta to ½ cup and meat servings to 2-3 ounces per day.

Diabetes:

Certain foods we eat are changed into glucose (sugar) and carried in the blood stream to our body's cells, where it is used for energy. Insulin, a hormone made by the pancreas helps drive this glucose into the cells. Those with diabetes either do not make enough insulin (Type I) or what they make does not work well enough (Type II), and therefore the glucose in the blood stream stays high. This can cause extreme thirst, blurred vision, tiredness, constant hunger, numbness or tingling in the hands or feet, dry skin, poor wound healing, or repeated infections. If left untreated over time, there can be damage to the eyes, heart and kidney.

a) Type I (juvenile) diabetes affects children, teens and young adults who are usually of normal weight. The cause is unknown but believed to involve autoimmune, genetic, and/or environmental factors. The body's immune system attacks and destroys certain cells in the pancreas (B cells), preventing the patients' ability to make insulin. Supplemental inject able insulin is needed to maintain the delicate balance between sugar in the blood and that taken into the body's cells. Appropriately scheduled dietary needs (especially carbohydrates), required insulin management, and essential exercise programs are the treatments necessary for this disorder. Talking with a dietary counselor is required since strict adherence to timing of meals and insulin injections are paramount.

b) Type II diabetics is a serious disease, so if you have it, you need to get serious. Most patients are older, and/or overweight with sedentary or inactive lifestyles. Other risk factors include race; namely African-American, Hispanic-Latino, American-Indian, and Asian-Pacific Islanders are significant more predisposed to this disease than any other race. Diabetic patients are also at greater risk for high blood pressure, high cholesterol, heart disease, and high-risk pregnancies. Though the pancreas produces insulin, it does not work as well or is not enough to meet the body's needs. Follow a physician-directed diet, exercise, take prescribed medications and lose some weight. There is no getting around it, and having a diet coke with a piece of cake is not a diet!

Though a majority of Type II diabetic patients are overweight, most recently Type II diabetes has been targeting another group of women -those who are fit! The National Institute of Health states that about 15 percent of people with Type II diabetes are not overweight. Jimmy Bell, M.D., a molecular imaging expert, has identified a condition called TOFI—thin outside, fat inside. "Neglecting exercise and regulating weight through food choices alone without breaking a sweat, stress, yo-yo diets and lack of exercise are culprits for developing this condition," claims Betel Hatipoglu, M.D., an endocrinologist at the Cleveland Clinic. He believes when you lose weight through dieting, you also lose muscle. Then when an appropriate weight management program is not maintained, you regain that weight. However, you gain only fat, not the muscle. In other words, "yo-yo dieters" lose the muscle needed to burn fat and control blood sugar, which can increase the likelihood of developing Type II diabetes.

THE DIABETIC DIET:

General recommendations

There are three basic food groups: fats, proteins, and carbohydrates. In diabetes, it is important to have all three of these food groups included in the diet, but in moderation and proportional. The Diabetes Food Pyramid is used as a guide for the diabetic diet and bases these food groups on carbohydrate and protein content. It splits foods into six groups and serving sizes, encouraging more food choices from the bottom of the pyramid (grains, beans, and starchy vegetables). These food groups are loaded with vitamins, minerals, fiber, and healthy carbohydrates. There is a misconception that diabetes is caused by the sugar you eat, but it can be affected by most foods, especially carbohydrates. Carbohydrates serve as the main energy source in the diet Most of our carbohydrates come from starch, milk and fruit, while some are found in vegetables. Carbohydrates are not really found in meats and fats, however despite this, they can contribute significantly to the calorie count. Make sure to choose from "healthy" carbohydrates: fruits, vegetables, whole grains, beans, peas, lentils, whole-wheat flour and wheat bran. Keep dairy products low-fat.

General recommendations necessitate that 45 - 65 percent of the day's total calories come from carbohydrates, 15 - 20 percent from protein, and 25 to 35 percent from fat. Saturated fats should be limited to less than 7 percent, and Trans fats should be completely avoided. Total cholesterol intake should be less than 200 mg per day, fiber 25-30 grams per day, and sodium less than 1500 mg per day.

Ginseng raises pancreatic insulin secretion and increases your cell's ability to burn glucose, which gives you more energy. Basil has antioxidants, rosemarinic acid and eugenol, which lowers cortisol and protects pancreas from damage. Vitamin D and calcium control pancreatic release of insulin. Avoid beef, hot dogs, sausage, high-fat dairy products, red meats, egg yolks, shellfish, liver and bacon. Monounsaturated and polyunsaturated fats like soybean, corn or extra virgin olive oil are better. Stay away from saturated fats (butter, coconut and palm oils) and Trans fats (processed snacks, baked goods, shortening and stick margarines). While these are some useful basic guidelines, it is very important to consult with a registered dietician who can explain how to measure food portions, count calories, and use the exchange program (groups foods into categories that have similar affect on blood sugar) and Glycemic index. Pay attention to portion sizes and fiber amounts. Education, practice, and assistance from a dietitian on understanding exchange planning diabetic diet management strategies. Always stay consistent. If weight is not an issue, a well-balanced diet is still needed. Exercise is good for everyone. Sometimes insulin is required and other times this type of diabetes is managed with oral medication. Either way, follow the advice of your health provider.

Hyperthyroid

Hyperthyroid disease, the thyroid gland produces too much thyroid hormone. This hormone controls your metabolism, or how fast food is broken down for energy. Patients often complain of feeling nervous, moody, weak, warm, sweaty, or tired. They may also experience weight loss, irregular menstrual cycles, difficulty breathing, a fast or irregular heartbeat, or hair that begins to get soft or fall out.

DIET:

Diet choices and healthy eating are important because women with hyperthyroid disorders often lose weight. It is important to maintain a healthy weight but not at the expense of eating unhealthy, fat laden foods. Most women with a moderately active lifestyle will consume 2,000-2,500 calories/day. If you are having difficulty maintaining weight, increase the amount of calories you consume each day, usually by 500-1,000 calories until you reach a healthy weight, then cut back to what you need to maintain your weight.

Your diet should include lean white meats and healthy fats, which are found in nuts, cheese, and dark chocolate. Good carbohydrate sources include whole grains, vegetables and fruit. A daily diet should always include strawberries, blueberries or raspberries. They are rich in antioxidants and good for your immune system.

Goitrogens, like broccoli, cauliflower, brussel sprouts, cabbage, mustard kale turnips rape seed soy and pine nuts, interfere suppress the amount of thyroid hormone the body produces, and are helpful in those with hyperthyroid, who make too much hormone. These are great, however, they should be used in moderation.

Certain foods can actually worsen hyperthyroid symptoms. Excessive iodine intake, found in large quantities of iodized table salt or shellfish, pushes the thyroid gland to make more thyroid hormone. Avoid these as well as eggs, mayonnaise, dairy products like whole milk, certain cheeses (i.e.: cheddar) and yogurt. Other high sources of iodine are iodine-rich plants (i.e.: kelp), sea bass, haddock, cod and perch, artichokes and spinach. In addition, avoid processed meats, like sausage and hamburger, that may contain the thyroid gland of the animal.

Avoid aspartame, a non-caloric artificial sweetener that some experts claim high doses can lead to hyperthyroidism. Brand names for this product are Equal-Measure, Equal and NutraSweet.

Hypothyroid

In hypothyroid disease, the thyroid gland produces too little thyroid hormone and is underactive, slowing down your metabolism. Symptoms can include fatigue, memory loss, depression, unexplained weight gain and hoarseness. Patients also complain of muscle weakness or aches, increased sensitivity to cold, dry skin, irregular menstrual periods, thin hair, constipation, or slow heart rate.

A healthy diet for someone with hypothyroidism would include whole grains, plenty of fruits and vegetables, and a good supply of seafood and other lean protein. Other good diet options include fiber, beans, rice and other grains, whole wheat and oatmeal. These foods make you feel full, help with weight lose, and improve constipation. Eat between four and five small meals of 300 calories each, instead of 3 big meals, and spread them throughout the day. Add Selenium, a trace mineral that acts as an antioxidant. It is essential for converting T4, the thyroid hormone your body produces, into T3, its active form. Good sources of Selenium include Brazil nuts, sunflower seeds, walnuts, raisins and wheat germ. Most of your carbohydrates should come from fruits and vegetables and drinking lots of water (a good idea for anyone, not just those suffering with hypothyroid disease).

Some doctors recommend the "Zone" diet, which balances out your insulin reaction.

The diet calls for more fruit and vegetables and less pasta, bread and other starches, and a small amount of lean protein through the day,

In contrast with hyperthyroidism, patients with hypothyroidism should avoid Goitrogens. As previously mentioned, Goitrogens include broccoli, cauliflower, brussel sprouts, cabbage, mustard kale turnips, grape seed, soy, and pine nuts. These will interfere with iodine uptake and may further suppress an already underactive thyroid gland.

Alzheimer's disease

Alzheimer's disease, commonly known as Alzheimer's, is the most common form of dementia. This disease progressively affects memory, thinking and behavior. Many confuse this disease with part of the normal aging process, but it is not. This disorder causes a progressive brain degeneration and dysfunction. Symptoms can start with short-term memory loss and later develop into confusion, irritability, aggression, mood swings, trouble with language, and eventually long-term memory loss. The deterioration of these intellectual abilities becomes serious enough to interfere with one's daily life. Ultimately the patient withdraws from family and society. Over time, bodily functions are lost, and death is imminent. The average life expectancy following diagnosis is approximately seven years. There is no cure for the disease, but patients who have mental stimulation, an exercise program, and balanced diet have shown slowing of the disease's progression.

Alzheimer's Improvement/Prevention Diet:

Although researchers have differing views of dietary changes for the improvement and prevention of Alzheimer's, recent research suggests a reduction of your intake of foods high in fat and cholesterol, and an increase in your intake of foods with high levels of naturally occurring antioxidant levels as they may protect against brain cell damage. Generally, these foods include dark-skinned fruits, like prunes, raisins, blueberries, blackberries, strawberries, Gogi berries, raspberries, plums, oranges, red grapes and cherries, and certain vegetables, like kale, spinach, brussel sprouts, alfalfa sprouts, broccoli, beets, red bell pepper, onion, corn and eggplant. Beneficial omega-3 fatty acids, as found in cold water fish like halibut, mackerel, salmon, trout and tuna, also help the brain transmit information between cells. Foods rich in curry may also be beneficial as it contains curcumin, an Indian spice researchers believe may help prevent memory loss as the spice has been shown to clear amyloid plaques deposited in the brain which has been linked to memory loss. Finally, it is important to keep your diet rich in fiber like whole grains. Whole grains are a main source of fuel for the brain, which is needed for energy, stabilization of blood sugar levels, and digestion.

Other good sources of antioxidants can be found in vitamin E, vitamins E and C together, vitamin B12 and folate. Eat foods rich in Vitamin C, such as orange and grapefruit juice, peaches, papaya, cranberries, strawberries, peppers, broccoli, brussel sprouts, and Vitamin E (almonds, pecans, sunflower seeds, paprika, chili powder, almonds, pine nuts, peanuts, oregano, basil, apricots, olive, spinach, and avocado). Most of these foods also reduce the risk of heart disease and stroke.

As always, in addition to a healthy and selective diet, and supplements of Vitamins found in fruits and vegetables, make sure to exercise in moderation and keep in touch with friends and family to keep the brain stimulated.

Is She a Nurse or a Curse?

I lay in bed
Silently in pain
I've been here for days
But you don't know my name

Sometimes I make
A simple request
It might be a headache
I'm not at my best

The fear of not knowing
What's happened to me?
Keeps a funeral silence
Around constantly

Just seeing a smile
Or a comforting touch
Spreads a peaceful blanket
That would mean so much

But you just keep writing
On a chart with my name
It's just paper and ink
We're not both the same

I'm cold and I'm tired
Without faith you see
Why push the knife deeper
And deeper in me

If we could exchange
You'd be in this bed
And eyes would flow tears
For things that are said

So dig down deep
You may find the part
Get acquainted again
That once was your heart

Arthritis

Arthritis is a chronic inflammatory disease that causes pain, limited movement or swelling in one or more joints. Most damage occurs when cartilage breaks down, causing bones to rub together. Arthritis typically affects joints in the fingers, wrists, knees, back, hips and elbows. There is no cure, but one can prevent the condition from worsening by maintaining a normal weight, which can reduce stress on joints and ease pain, exercising, and engaging in positive therapies, like whirlpool and physical therapy.

There two major types of arthritis currently afflicting people. Both can have similar symptoms but different causes. Rheumatoid arthritis result when the body is attacked by its own immune system, which Osteoarthritis can result from age, trauma or daily wear and tear affecting the joints.

Diet:

Foods that are known to reduce inflammation may improve arthritis symptoms. Fruits rich in Boron, a mineral known to nourish the material that builds stronger cartilage and joint tissue, like raisins, prunes and almonds, and vitamin C, such as citrus type fruits, kiwifruit, peaches and oranges have been known reduce inflammation. Other fruits and vegetables, like sweet potatoes, carrots, butternut squash, apricots, cantaloupe, pumpkin, corn, red peppers and tangerines, containing Beta carotene, may help reduce the arthritis related symptoms. Fruits and vegetables containing Beta carotene are typically deep red, orange, yellow, or green in color. Beta carotene contains beta-cryptoxanthin, which protects cells from the damaging effects of free radicals and provides a great source of vitamin A. Some studies suggest that SAM-e, especially when taken in conjunction with vitamin B-12, B-6, and folate, works as well as some over-the-counter pain medications. The body uses Sam_E to make certain chemicals that control pain.

Additionally, whole-wheat products, like rye, bulgar, oats, quinoa, brown rice, wild rice and barley, contain ample amounts of omega-3, essential fatty acids, and selenium, all antioxidant cell protector. Cold water fish, like sardines, mackerel, trout and salmon, are also abundant in omega-3. Other sources rich in omega-3 include soybeans, walnuts, pumpkin and oils like extra virgin olive, flaxseed, canola and sunflower. Moreover, adding ginger, flaxseed, cumin, and/or turmeric to curries, soups, or stews has also been shown to decreased inflammation.

Certain foods may worsen symptoms and thus should be avoided. Most foods containing Omega-6 fatty acids, which is found in meat and poultry, may aggravate arthritic symptoms. A vegetarian or vegan diet has been shown to reduce arthritic symptoms. However gamma linolenic acid (GLA), an omega-6 fatty acid found in evening primrose oil, black currant oil and borage oil supplements, is a substance the body uses to make anti-inflammatory agents, so it can actually reduce arthritic symptoms. Avoid nightshade vegetables, like potatoes, eggplant, most peppers and tomatoes. Omit saturated fats found in full-fat dairy products, butter, fatty meats and baked foods. Acid foods like sugar, coffee, red meat, most grains, nuts and citrus fruits, should also be avoided.

Osteoporosis

Bone tissue is constantly in the process of remodeling, which involves the simultaneous building up and breaking down of bone. As one becomes older, an imbalance in this process develops and more bone is broken down than is built. This causes existing bone to become soft and susceptible to osteoporosis, a disease causing bones to become fragile and more likely to fracture. The hips, spine and wrist are most often affected.

Diet:

To avoid Osteoporosis, a diet with a healthy supply of fruits and vegetables, which will provide the necessary phytochemicals, minerals and vitamins to support bone growth, is beneficial. Food rich in Calcium and Vitamin D are also needed and can slow down bone loss. Good sources of calcium are green leafy vegetables, baked beans, bony fish, dried fruit and low-fat milk, cheese and yogurt. Vitamin D can be found in fortified milk, egg yolks, saltwater fish, liver, and supplements. Get out in the sun too, as this increase Vitamin D production. Other beneficial vitamins and minerals include magnesium, vitamin A, vitamin D, vitamin B6and vitamin K are necessary for calcium absorption. Magnesium can be found in dried herbs such as coriander, chives, spearmint, dill, sage and basil. So, sprinkle, sprinkle, sprinkle.

To lessen the progression of bone loss, reduce your intake of red meat, chocolate and caffeine. Excess salt, sodas, deli turkey, ham and hot dogs also cause bone loss and should be avoided. Limit salt to 2,000 milligrams (mg) or one teaspoon a day. Exercise, especially weight bearing, and maintain a normal weight. Thin, Caucasian women are at greater risk, therefore if menopausal talk to your health care provider about available bone supportive therapies.

Asthma:

Asthma is a chronic inflammatory disease that affects the airways of the lungs and makes breathing difficult. This inflammation (swelling) also makes airways more sensitive, especially to irritants like pollen, dust, and smoke and pet dander. During an asthma attack, the muscles surrounding the airways contract, air passages swell, and oxygen exchange is reduced. Symptoms include wheezing, coughing, chest tightness and trouble breathing, especially early in the morning or at night. When symptoms become worse, patients can develop an asthma attack. This can severely block the lungs ability to exchange oxygen, often leading to hospitalization.

Asthma Prevention Diet:

Foods with anti-inflammatory properties may help reduce asthma symptoms or incidence of attacks. Add plenty of fresh fruits and vegetables to your diet. Antioxidants like beta carotene and vitamins C and E, reduce the number of free radicals that can cause swelling, irritation, and overall damage to those cells lining the lung's airways. Vitamin D which is found in milk, eggs, and natural sunlight, which increases the body's production vitamin D, also reduces asthma symptoms and incidence of attacks. Foods rich in omega-3 fatty acids like salmon, tuna, and sardines are also beneficial. Some researchers advocate for the Mediterranean diet, a diet high in nuts and fruits like grapes, apples, and tomatoes.

Certain foods should be avoided, as it may worsen asthma symptoms. Avoid Trans fats, omega-6 fatty acids and saturated fats, particularly those found in some margarine, saturated vegetable and partially hydrogenated oils and processed foods. Dairy products can increase mucus production, further clogging lung passages, making breathing difficult. Eliminate or reduce milk products, animal protein and fried foods. Avoid sulfites which are often used as a preservative found in wine, dried fruits, pickles, and fresh and frozen shrimp. If you are known to have problems with any foods, avoid them.

Lupus

Lupus is an inflammatory disease where the body begins to attack itself, often involving the kidney, heart, blood, and muscle, and the nervous, respiratory and gastrointestinal systems. Those affected may complain of difficulty breathing, visual disturbances, and may be at greater risk for cancer and infections. Emphasis should be on foods that are fresh, natural, and reduce inflammation.

Diet to reduce Lupus related symptoms:

Diets rich in fruits, vegetables that are high in antioxidants, substances known to protect against cell and tissue damage, whole grains, organic produce, and hormone-free animal products, especially low fat and lean meats like turkey, chicken and lamb, should be encouraged. Plant-based diets that are low in calories, fat and cholesterol are also suggested. Moreover, the American College of Rheumatology has found omega-3 fish oils improve lupus symptoms. Good sources are salmon, sardines, herring and mackerel. Polyunsaturated oils are better than saturated ones. Further, since patients with lupus are often on corticosteroids, a medication that weakens bone strength, diets with foods rich in calcium, a mineral necessary for the growth and maintenance of strong teeth and bones, are recommended. Calcium-rich foods are low-fat milk, cheese or yogurt and the vegetables turnip, mustard, dandelion greens, collards, and Kale.

Dried herbs, like celery seed, dried thyme, dill, marjoram, basil, sage, oregano, sesame and flax seeds, are great seasonings that are high in calcium, and that allow you to put down the salt. These can be added to meats, soups, salads or a favorite recipe. Foods rich in vitamin D, like fish, mushrooms, eggs and sweet potatoes help increase calcium absorption. Also look for foods fortified with Vitamin D like orange juice and cereals.

Certain foods should also be avoided in order to reduce symptoms which may promote painful inflammation and increase flare-ups. Foods such as, nightshade vegetables, like potatoes, tomatoes, peppers and eggplant, Tabasco, sweet and hot peppers, paprika and cayenne peppers, as well as fried and processed foods, saturated fats and soy products promote painful symptoms.

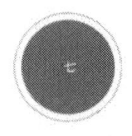

Slowly I turn
Step by step
Inch by inch
Deeper and deeper
Ouch....

CHAPTER SEVEN
My GYN Exam

Question: What's a gynecologist?

Answer: A man you don't have to ask is it in.

An alternate definition would be, "A specialist who has completed an approved Ob/Gyn residency training program." We should add, "...and renders quality medical services, accurate treatment and expected respect to women when evaluating their health care needs...." So what happened to Mary?

A spring ambiance complimented the friendly flow of patients in and out of the busy doctor's office, which lay quietly nestled between flocks of tall oaks. Ambience personified, Currier could not have described it better to Ives. Inside, the office was bustling with activity. Some patients were scattered amongst the friendly chatter while others found quiet comfort in reading the accessible magazines. "Mrs. Chamberlain, the doctor will see you now," chanted a friendly nurse's voice. Individually, she led anxiously waiting patients towards their respective evaluating room, her starched white serving as a directing beacon.

While passing a neatly curtain framed window, the nurse stopped abruptly, "There it is again!" The shadow of a partially cloaked '89 Ford Escort peaked amongst the arboresque background. She had seen this same car similarly parked on several previous occasions but the occupant never came inside. Then after a few minutes, just as mysteriously, the car would slowly pull away.

Who knew that seated inside that car was fear? Her name was Mary but that only identified a shell whose spirit abandoned long ago. Spiraled fingers tenaciously strangled a steering wheel tear stained. Mary could only tolerate brief glimpses into an imprisoned past; finding no unlocking keys in the present.

At the time, she was just a little girl, shy of ten years old. Tom was her neighborhood friend. They did everything together but her guardian grandma just misunderstood. Ruled by old and deep-rooted values that believed boys kept away from girls, an unwritten rule which substituted for contraception.

Despite Mary's pleas of unbroken virginity, her grandmother needed confirmation. It still seemed like yesterday, not thirty years ago. Dragged into that ruined, antiquated musky shack masquerading as a medical facility to see the doctor, but that was the worth of the southern poor. Mary begged, "Don't leave me alone!" However, the doctor insisted. Slowly and gentle at first, he guided her feet into the stirrups. That was his last gentle touch. Tears began to carve into Mary's face, as flashbacks appeared of hands too big that should not touch her there. Thirty years later the battle still rages inside.

It was only because of her friendly and concerned psychiatrist that Mary even agreed to see a gynecologist. "A Pap test is very important to look for cancer and you have never had one," he pleaded. "There is a new female doctor in the area, and I think you will like her." So Mary had been practicing going to her appointment for weeks, bravely driving her car to the *gynecologist's office, sitting there an unobstructed minute, then pulling away.*

Now today was different; it was the day of her appointment. Mary took a deep breath and mustered up some buried confidence, knowing her own health was more important than a damaging past.

Then she quietly drove away.

The ANNUAL GYN EXAM is vital to assist women in maintaining their health. It should include a detailed history, complete physical exam, and testing based on age recommendations. Knowing the basic details of these components will help you better understand, prepare, and ensure a proper and complete evaluation.

Detailed History

Below is historical information your doctor will need, especially if seeing you for the first time. Review and write down this information before your visit, take your time and make sure it is complete.

I. GYN HISTORY

A. LMP: (last menstrual period)

- What age did you start your first cycle?
- How long does your cycle last?
- How many days are between each cycle?
- Do you have a history of normal cycles?
- If abnormal, what is your bleeding pattern?
- Do you have any bleeding between your cycles?
- Can you have a period every two weeks or skip whole months?

- Is there heavy bleeding or severe pain?

- Do you have symptoms associated with your cycle such as headache, cramps, abnormal pain or bloating?

Do you have any symptoms of PMS? (Irritability, anxiety, breast pain, water retention or mood swings)

Initiation of the menstrual cycle starts around age twelve (11y.o. -14y.o.). It may be irregular in the beginning, sometimes taking years to develop into a normal pattern. An average time or interval between two menstrual cycles is usually 21 – 40 days (average 28 days). The first day of the cycle is the first day of bleeding and can last 1- 9 days (average 5 days). Irregular bleeding, especially in a woman's earlier years and after the cycle has become established can have multiple causes. These can include a hormonal imbalance called dysfunctional uterine bleeding (DUB), uterine leiomyomas (fibroids), unexpected pregnancy, thyroid disease, sexually transmitted infections (STI's) and polycystic ovarian disease.

Peri-menopause or climacteric is a time when the menstrual cycles should get lighter, further apart and eventually go away. Symptoms associated with this time of change also include anxiety, irritability, insomnia, mood swing, migraine headaches, memory loss, hot flashes, depression and loss of sexual desire. Women can experience physical changes such as sensitive/dry skin, smaller breast, bladder problems (unable to hold urine), dryness and itching in the vaginal area. Menopause means you have stopped your periods for one year and the average age is fifty-one.

Irregular cycles, abnormal spotting or heavy bleeding needs attention. This can consist of a personal examination, various labs, radiology test or possible surgical evaluations by a health provider. In women over 40, there is more of a cancer concern with abnormal vaginal bleeding than in younger women. An endometrial sampling allows acquiring tissue samples from the lining of the uterus (womb) that is sent to pathology. This can be done in the office, similar to having a Pap test, with mild-moderate cramping. In addition, a pelvic ultrasound can evaluate the thickness of that lining, the size of the uterus (womb) and examine the ovaries.

B. PAP, STI's and CONTRACEPTION

- Date of your last pelvic exam and Pap smear. Were either abnormal?

- If abnormal, were any tests, procedures or follow-up instructions given?

- Do you have a history of an abnormal Pap smear? If so, when?

- Do you have a history of any sexual infections (like Gonorrhea, Chlamydia, Herpes, Syphilis, HIV, Human Papilloma Virus (HPV) ...) or PID (pelvic infections)?

- What is your sexual history, gender preference (if comfortable) and number of sexual partners?

- What type of contraception have you used now or in the past? List them, names, dates and duration used.

- Did you have any problems taking contraception?
- Are you interested in any particular contraceptive or information on contraception?

Choose carefully your contraception. Combination birth control pills, patches, and rings contain synthetic estrogen and progesterone hormone components. Newer products may have a greater risk of complications compared with older products, especially blood clots. Obesity, smoking, diabetes and/or personal/strong family history of heart disease, blood clots or stroke may be risk factors for taking the estrogen in the combination pills. Progesterone –only contraception lacks estrogen and includes Depo-Provera, Norplant or the Mini-Pills. You should not take contraceptive pills if you are over 35 and smoke cigarettes.

IUD's are devices inserted in the uterus (womb) and can have up to 10 years of pregnancy protection, depending on the type used. After insertion, you should check its attached string monthly. The IUD may be acceptable for older patients, those with single sex partners and completed families.

Condoms reduce the risk of sexual infections but those from animal intestines (lambskin) are thin and may not protect completely against A.I.D.S., Herpes, Chlamydia or Hepatitis B. Latex condoms better shield against these infection.

Tubal ligation procedures provide permanent contraception. Some are performed in an operating room or Surgi-center through an incision on the lower abdomen or a scope placed right below the navel. Others can be done in an office setting where plugs are placed in the openings of the fallopian tubes through a scope introduced into the uterus via the vagina (Essure). If making this decision, it should be viewed as a permanent solution. Some of these procedures can be reversed but the success depends on the type of procedure done and if there is any damage to a woman's pelvic organs, fallopian tubes and/or uterus.

II. OBSTETRICAL HISTORY

Each pregnancy experience is important. Try to access as much complete detail as possible. Get your records if needed, especially if complicated.

You need to list each pregnancy, dates of delivery, type of delivery, length of labor, baby's weight, sex and Apgar score. Also list outcomes and any pregnancy complications. Include name, address and phone number of delivery provider and hospital. Include miscarriages, abnormal, molar or tubal pregnancies.

III. GENERAL MEDICAL HISTORY

Are you being treated for now or in the past, any medical problems, especially high blood pressure, asthma, TB, bronchitis, lupus, diabetes, psychiatric disorders, rheumatic fever and/or heart disease? All past medical problems are important. BE SURE TO GET A COPY OF PAST MEDICAL RECORDS and allow 2-6 weeks to get them in the mail.

You can call the office and pick up your medical records in person if needed sooner. A signature is required on all medical information releases and sometime charges are incurred. Make sure to ask for progress notes, consultations, labs, radiology reports, hospital discharge summaries and operative reports. It is ILLEGAL for this information to be withheld from you.

Allergies

Are you allergic to any medications?
List them and what type of reactions you have had.

Medication

Are you currently taking any medications?
What is the name, dose, how often do you take it and how long have you been on the medication?

Always list over the counter medications and herbal supplements. Chronic use of even over the counter medications can cause health problems. Excess Tylenol is related to liver problems and NSAIDS (Motrin, Advil, and Alleve) to ulcers and bowel disturbances.

Smoking

Do you smoke cigarettes? How much, how often and how long?

Smoking kills silently. It increases the risk of lung cancer, bronchitis, and emphysema and may contribute to heart disease. Nicotine products plus counseling can be a helpful approach to quit smoking and women do better than men.

Alcohol

Do you drink alcohol? How much and how often, be truthful. Excess use can lead to liver and brain problems.

Hospitalizations/Surgery:

You should list type of any surgery or reasons for hospitalization. Include dates, doctors/hospitals involved including addresses and phone numbers. Also list any diagnosis and/or complications

Lab/X-Ray/Ultrasounds/Other Radiology studies

Make sure to get reports of all evaluations.

IV. FAMILY MEDICAL HISTORY

Certain medical problems run in families placing you at risk. If you are not sure, talk to relatives. List disorders like who have had or has high blood pressures, cancer, diabetes, heart disease and/or genetic disorders) that may affect family members.

V. SOCIAL HISTORY

What are your marital status, occupation, educational level, living environment and any social problems?

Social services departments are located in most hospitals and health clinics. In addition, private offices may have referral numbers for such services. This can be helpful in emergencies and locating services, you may be entitled. Don't be afraid to ask.

If you are seeing your doctor for a problem or just an annual GYN exam, you should still fill out a complete history if not previously recorded.

IV. REASON FOR VISIT

Common chief complaints

If there is a problem, it is important to describe the problem in detail.

Here are some common gyn-related problems.

PAIN:

Where is it is located?
Is it constant or does it come and go?
Does it radiate to other areas?
How long has it been there?
Are there other associated signs/symptoms like fever, chills, nausea, vomiting, constipation or diarrhea?

Do certain things make it better or worse? (eating, breathing, changing positions, etc.)

DISCHARGE:

How long has it been there?
What color is the discharge?
Does it itch or have an odor to it?

Any fever, chills or abdominal pain?
Does your sexual partner have any symptoms?
Any history of sexual infections?

BLADDER/BOWEL

Are there any bladder problems?(pain with passing urine, going too often, voiding at night or passing urine with a cough or sneeze)

Are there any bowel problems?
(constipation, diarrhea, bloody stools, indigestion)
Is there a previous personal or family history of bowel or bladder problems?

An additional copy of all this information should be kept in a file at home labeled "personal medical information". Software is also available to help you better store personal medical histories if you are computer savvy, like Minerva Health Manager, My Life Record and Medefile.

My Gynecologist

Slowly passed the midnight sky, ticking away at the wee morning hours. A desolate train station decorated the background below. Although partially cloaked by a tenacious fog, the lack of human presence was obvious. Blinking railroad-crossing lights seen in the distance remained the stations only identification. Pitter and then patter sounds emerged with soft footsteps heard in the background. The secluded train station and these sounds were companions for a few seconds before the silent figure emerged.

There stood a reflection of womanhood, depressed by too many emotional roller coasters. Her frail body smothered by the oversized trench coat and a brim that partially covered her face. "He's in and out so fast." The burdened words rolled past a solemn tongue. The sullen shadow continued walking alone, identified momentarily by a lit cigarette that hung from partially pressed lips. Following a deep, sucking breath, these words followed. "I don't think he ever looked at my face." Silent tears fell but she knew they were there. "That thing is cold when he puts it in!" Just recanting brought a sudden chill.

No, it's not a man I'm talking about." "It's my gynecologist.

V. ANNUAL GYN EXAM

This is probably on the top of many women's dreaded things to do list. However, it is an important exam, requires comfortableness on your part and an understanding from your provider. This exam should still have essential components of a complete physical, not just a quick thrust of the speculum into the vagina of a partially clad nervously freezing patient.

Your vital signs should be taken and recorded, at least a blood pressure, weight and pulse. Hypertension or high blood pressure may have no symptoms and an abnormal pulse can pick up thyroid problems or abnormalities in the heart's rate or rhythm. A weight is checked at each visit, as excessive gain or loss of weight may uncover other hidden medical complications like thyroid disorders, hidden cancers, HIV or bowel-related problems.

Prior to the pelvic exam, a general physical examination is performed to at least check the breast, lungs, heart and abdomen. Additional areas may also be examined based on the thoroughness of the examiner.

Physical

General appearance: Do you look normal or not? Is your skin healthy? Are you mentally alert? Are there signs of severe weight loss or gain? Any signs of distress like difficulty breathing, sweating or shortness of breath? Can you walk and stand without problems?

HEENT: Evaluation of the head (shape and contour), ears (inner and external ear), eyes (check pupils for reaction to light), neck (check thyroid gland), and throat (look for any redness, swelling or discharge on tonsils. Also check inside of the mouth).

Lungs: Listen with a stethoscope to the lungs to see if the breath sounds are normal or if any abnormal breath sound can be heard like wheezes or crackles. That might indicate asthma, bronchitis or other lung disorders.

Cardiovascular: The heart sounds are also listened to with a stethoscope making sure there is a regular rate and rhythm. Abnormal or extra heart sounds and irregular beats may indicate heart disease.

Breast: Examination of both breast including the breast tissue, areola (nipple) and auxiliary tail (amount of breast tissue that extends into the underarm). Self-breast examination should be reviewed if requested and literature given if available. A baseline mammogram is suggested at age 40, every 1-2 years, between the ages 40-50 and every year after the age of 50 by most authorities.

Abdomen: The abdomen is felt and examined in all quadrants (upper and lower abdomen) for any pain, tenderness, guarding or masse. Tapping the abdomen helps to look for fluid. Listens to bowel sounds and check liver size.

Extremities: Examination of the hands and feet to make sure there is no cyanosis (blue discoloration), edema (swelling) or clubbing (change in fingers, nail beds are soft and appear curved.) This may indicate decreased oxygen.

Back: Check curvature of spine to see if normal or any signs of scoliosis (spine has abnormal curve). Tap on lower back to check kidneys.

Neuro: Review of nerves, reflexes and muscle strength. Also evaluate mental status.

Pelvic Exam

A Pap test can be difficult for some women, especially those who are young, infrequently sexually active, same sex partnered or understandably nervous. There are some ways to make it easier. Take an over the counter pain medicine like Tylenol, Aleve or Advil as directed before and after the exam if there are no allergies.

During this exam, the woman is asked to lie back, put her feet in the stirrups and come down to the edge of the table. The examiner should inspect the outer area of the female genitals for any abnormalities, discolorations or moles. Any mole in that area may need a biopsy to rule out cancer no matter what it looks like or what age you are. The Bartholin glands that lie on each side of the lower vulva are checked for any signs of infection or enlargement.

The speculum is then introduced into the vagina. It only appears to be as large as the room you are in. However, speculums do come in various sizes, small, medium and large. You can request a smaller size especially if you have difficulty with the exam. Other types that insert easier are nasal, pediatric graves, Huffman-Graves or Pederson speculums. You can request that one of these special speculums is available when you make your appointment.

The examiner will then look inside the vagina for any abnormalities. They can only see the walls of the vagina and the cervix, or lower end of the uterus (womb). A Pap test is then taken. Cells are collected from the cervix and sent to a pathologist to look for cancer or precancerous changes, better treated when detected early. We know that cervical cancer is very slow growing, and in many, the abnormal pre-cancer changes (dysplasia) can be present for many years before a true cancer develops. But in others, it may develop more rapidly than expected. The National Cancer Institute estimates 12,170 new cases of cervical cancer with 4,220 deaths. This is still a concerning disease. Keep up with your PAP smears.

In November 2009, the American College of Obstetrics and Gynecology changed the recommendations for PAP smears, a revolutionary test that has significantly decreased the risk of cervical cancer in women. Now, a woman has her first Pap smear at age 21 unless there has been a previously abnormal pap smear.

Those 21 to 30 can be screened every two years instead of annually.

If age 30 or older with 3 negative consecutive PAP smears, the test can be extended to every three years.

Women who have had a hysterectomy for non-cancerous reasons like chronic pain, fibroids (leiomyomas) or abnormal bleeding do not need a Pap smear if the cervix was removed.

If you have had a hysterectomy but still have your cervix or your hysterectomy was for pre-cancer changes (dysplasia even if your cervix was removed, you will need to continue routine Pap smears.

Cervical cancer screening with PAP smears can also be discontinued at age 65 or 70 if there have been three or more negative PAP smears in a row and no abnormal test results over the past 10 years.

Now there are even newer recommendations. The U.S. Preventive Services Task Force now has added, "For women ages 30 to 65 years who want to lengthen the screening interval, screening with a combination of cytology and human papillomavirus (HPV, suggest testing every 5 years."

What they didn't do is equate these new recommendations to how often you should see your doctor. Don't wait on potential problems or concerns because the annual Pap smear has been extended. It is still advised to visit your health provider once a year.

Certain women will need more frequent Pap test screening like those who have HIV, multiple sex partners, previous abnormal Pap test and those with immune system problems. Also, don't let your health insurance guide your access to a Pap smear. The traditional Pap test cost $20-40 and cells are placed on a traditional slide. The thin prep Pap cost $45-60, a little more because the cells collected for the test are placed in a liquid-based medium that gets rid of blood, mucus and debris. These cells are then easier to read for abnormalities.

HPV (Human Pappillomavirus) is a sexually transmitted virus that increases the risk of an abnormal Pap and certain strains have been related to cervical cancer. This fastidious virus has infiltrated the population, and has become the most common sexually transmitted disease. It affects 20 million Americans, with teens and adolescents at highest risk. HPV affects the mouth, throat and genital areas. It is passed through vaginal or anal sex, but also from oral sex, so be careful of those "friends with benefits" and the belief that oral sex is not really sex. Those infected with HPV can go on to develop genital or anal warts, but more serious, oral, anal, and as mentioned cervical cancer. Having the HPV vaccine does not change the Pap smear recommendations.

After the PAP is taken, you can be checked for infections, if requested or if an abnormal discharge is present. The provider can also look at the discharge under the microscope to diagnose local infections such as Trichmonas, Bacterial Vaginosis and Candida (Yeast). Cultures or urine samples can be checked for the sexual infections, Chlamydia and Gonorrhea.

Unfortunately, 80% of women and 20% of men may have no symptoms of these infections, acquired from a sexual partner. I encourage sexually active women to be checked once a year although this is not recommended unless under the age of 25 and insurance companies may not pay for them to be done electively. If these infections are present and not treated, many times with a simple antibiotic, they can spread and cause damage to the woman's reproductive organs. This can lead to chronic and poorly treated abdominal pain, infertility, PID (pelvic inflammatory disease) and possibly a need for a hysterectomy. It may be worth paying for this test once a year. Besides, what have you done for you lately?

Now the examiner will then do a bi-manual exam. One or two fingers are placed in the vagina and the other on the patient's lower abdomen. This is to check for the size/position of the uterus (womb) and size of the ovaries. Sometimes nodules associated with endometriosis can be felt as well as other pelvic masses like tubal pregnancies, ovarian masses and "chocolate cyst" from PID (pelvic inflammatory disease).

A rectal-vaginal exam may be needed in women over 40. For this exam, one finger is placed in the vagina and one in the rectum. The other hand is placed on the lower abdomen and the exam is completed as above. Stool guiac, a test for blood in the stools, can be done on stool from the rectal exam and results are given immediately. In addition, a colonoscopy is recommended for women over 50 and every 10 years unless there is a personal/family history of colon-rectal cancer that require more frequent testing.

I cannot stress the importance of being comfortable with your medical examiner. You scheduled an appointment, probably waited a bit and deserve the time it takes to do a proper exam.

Ask questions! If the response is not comfortable, trust your intuition and find another examiner. Don't unconsciously become another Mary. To have an exam does not help you is no different than not having an exam at all.

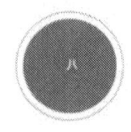

It's a curse to be in love
Because you can't cut out the pain
The feelings that you have
Are shot into your veins

They travel towards you soul
And occupy a space
Embedded so deep
They never erase

You tell yourself to let go
For many others are around
But in each you seek that Special One
And in them they are never found

So cherish what keeps you strong
Have faith along the way
For most of life peace will come
Except on Valentine's Day

CHAPTER EIGHT
Making Home, Family, Friends, Jobs, & Relationships Work

Relationships: Control the Madness

Relationships don't just not work; we work hard to make sure they don't. Oh, we are not aware of our contribution to the ultimate destruction of our relationships because we often fail to take any blame. However, we are all well aware of our partner's faults.

This is problematic because we can't change someone else's behavior, just our own. The true solution lay in asking: Are we doing what we can to make this relationship work? But before that, is this relationship worth it? A workable relationship has balance. It is imperative that both partners are contributing, not always equally, just always. So ask yourself, are you getting back in a relationship what you are putting into it? Without balance on both sides it may be destined to fail. No further discussion; find a new relationship.

Now some of us feel a relationship's importance becomes tallied on what our partner does gives and buys for us. Ultimately, chronic servitude doesn't add up to a suitable relationship, just that you have found a fool.

So start by taking a long look at the relationship you are in. I'll wait a minute, because some of you may need to look a little longer than others. After looking at your past relationships, determine your commitment level.

Read the two scenarios listed below. Which best fits you?

Scenario #1

- I am my own person, but would like to share my life with someone.

- I want to take time to find a relationship that works. I can be happy by myself.

- Being in a good relationship just takes me to another level.

Scenario #2

- I would rather be in a relationship instead of being alone.
- I just want to have children.
- Most of the good partners are already taken.
  I will always find a way to make my relationship happy.

If you identify more with Scenario #1, you are grounded and comfortable with yourself. Life is what motivates you; not dependence on a relationship. However, in your quest through life, a good relationship can add to your positivity, you are not willing to just settle for any relationship. Because you have found other things important in your life, you are willing to wait for the relationship that works for you. When you find it, you will be committed.

If you identify more with Scenario #2, you have preconceived your life and a relationship just becomes a place to fit it in. You are not independent, just traditional. Life is supposed to be structured, with a husband, kids and a picket fence. Anything less appears as defeat and appearances are paramount. You are probably a product of your upbringing which you have cloned into your current existence. Wait on a committed relationship until you have first had a chance to find yourself.

YOUR PAST: YOUR KEY TO A GREATER FUTURE

Imagine what a timesaver it would be if you could spend just a little time with someone and quickly know if they have what it takes to make a great relationship. This might sound impossible, but it's not. You can figure out what makes you desirable to others and, just as importantly, what will make one of them a good match for you. The keys lie in your past relationships. There is a high likelihood that you've had at least one romantic experience, even if your relationship experience is very limited. Take a trip down memory lane, starting with your first date. Write down the name of the person who asked you out. Then, make a list of answers to these questions:

- How did you meet?
- What was this special person like?
- What initially attracted you to each other?
- What did you do on your first date?
- Was it a good experience?
- Did you see each other again?
- Why or why not?
- How did the relationship end?
- Why?

If you have never been on a date in your life, think about any people you might have dated? Who were they and why didn't you ever make a connection with them?

Now, go through all your past significant relationships, and for each of them write down the answers to the same questions. If you haven't had any significant relationships, write down the names and particulars of people you have dated a few times, had a crush on, or were attracted to. The answer what happened to your relationship with these people.

Your Relationship History

Your tastes may have changed over time, but your basic personality and the types of people who attract you (and whom you attract) are probably the same. Perhaps all of your partners were emotionally needy. Perchance many were adventurous. Did most of your past partners have a good sense of humor or a positive, upbeat outlook? Did you see a history of physical violence, verbal abuse, and constant fighting? Were the people you dated unable to commit or unavailable?

Go back through your notes and select the top six assets (those you absolutely require from a partner) and the top six liabilities (things that you will never accept in a partner) and note those. Then, determine what assets and liabilities you bring to relationships that is valued or rejected by others. Armed with this information, you should be able to zone in more quickly on "your type" of potential new and better successful partner, as well as spot red flags in your date's past, personality, or values, which may signal that this person isn't a great candidate for a relationship with you.

Nevertheless, don't let go of your essence because you hit a bump in the road to relationship success. The world holds more than we can truly encompass, so don't try to understand it, and sometimes just accept things for what they are. When you venture into that vast abyss called life, it's like putting on a heavy coat adorned with complicated buttons. Some get fastened and some don't. We can't completely control the irritation of a workforce, impatience in our encounters, or nuisance of our associations. However, when we come home, we can take that coat off and leave it on the rack. Keep your home peaceful, and that sometimes takes a bit of work...but it's worth it. Don't worry... the coat will still be hanging there when you need to go out into the world again.

STRESSFULLY YOURS

Plop, plop, fizz, fizz... oh what a relief it isn't. The Schuyhill expressway is no place to be during rush hour. There is always ongoing construction, and nothing ever seems to get completed. They just seem to move from one part of the expressway to another.

Barbara glanced at the surrounding drivers. Traffic had been at a standstill for the past thirty minutes. What was everyone else trying to do to kill time? The couple in the blue gray Honda was arguing. A teenager, visible through her rear view mirror, was applying a third coat of make-up. Somewhere in the crowd was a car with New York license plates, introducing us all to Lil John's latest rap. Typical Philadelphia! Barbara took a deep breath, "I'll be glad when I get home."

It was different being a single professional woman. The promotion to editor of the Woman's Chronicle was superficial glory. To Barbara it meant more work and less personal time. Deadlines to meet, stories to proof, clients to appease; all requiring that painted on laugh.

"Why should Andy be surprised that I fell asleep during his company's dinner last week?" Barbara reminisced. "It's not easy to wake up and find your cheek in the French Onion Soup!" The familiar brown duplex was a welcome sight, as her green MGB Sports Coupe was carefully parked next to 1706. The neighborhood's quiescence gave Barbara a sense of relief from a hectic day. She hurried up the steps as visions of a "warm bubble bath" danced in her head. The key was barely in the door when the incessantly ringing phone began.

"Hello," Barbara gasped as she lunged for the phone, dropping her briefcase and spilling its contents. The deep husky voice on the other end could only be Andy. "Hi honey! Are you home?" "No," Barbara answered huffily. "I'm not home. I'm just standing here waiting for the bus and yes, I'm still mad..." Click. "If that phone rings one more time I'll scream," Barbara shouted as she violently flipped the switch to the answering machine. Ring...ring...click. The melodious voice of the answering service signaled that no one was available. "It's your mother," the caller identified," and turn off that machine because I know you're there...Hello, hello..." Click. Barbara moved toward the phone but hesitated. She didn't want to talk with anyone, not mother, and especially not Andy. A moment of peace, Barbara thought blissfully while running out the front door.

A light snow had just fallen. The Thomas Kindle-like Christmas serenity was never so prominent. Barbara could have climbed right into the sled and rode to grandma's house. Thoughts of the previous day sifted through her mind. She contemplated how different her life was, being a single professional woman. That requires elaboration. What people think your life should be and what it really is are different. Being single and professional are glorious only to those who are not. The stresses are sometimes unbearable, but the rewards are tremendous. You feel like lady justice trying to balance the scales with a blindfold on.

Herself blinded with thoughts of how hectic life had been, Barbara did not see the bright red eighteen-wheeler that zoomed past the intersection. There was not enough time to stop. The small compact MGB with its professional passenger remained helpless. All Barbara remembered was that she had the right of way, and the sound of steel crushing around her.

The room was completely dark except for a thin slit of light that peaked through the pink and green curtains. Barbara was drenched in sweat as she emerged from her worse nightmare. "What a dream!" She remained helpless. Her eyes were closed but she quickly opened them. The familiar surroundings of her bedroom were a welcome sight. Suddenly there was an appreciation for Andy...and her mother.

Stress - (Psychological) – "a condition typically characterized by symptoms of mental and physical tension or strain, as depression or hypertension, that can result from a reaction to a situation in which a person feels threatened, pressured," etc. (Webster's New World Dictionary)

Stress is an intangible enemy that conquers people by allowing us to unknowingly destroy ourselves. It removes the most precious thing we own, our peace of mind. Tension, anxiety, irritability and irrationality are often byproducts. Stress creates havoc with our job, family and personal relationships. We will stretch to unreasonable limits to maintain our livelihood and material possessions.

We are all aware of the hard work and sacrifices we've made to achieve our goals. One thing to remember is "if you didn't want it, you wouldn't have it." Don't frustrate yourself, waiting for someone to pat you on the back for a job well done. If it's that important to you, pat yourself on the back, or tell yourself that you did a great job on the tasks that you completed.

Allowing the stresses of life to get the best of you is like the fortresses that surround castles. Don't become a victim and shut yourself off. The way we handle stress dictates its effect on our lives. We should maintain and strengthen our true self.

We have all experienced disappointments in our lives and on the job. Work related stressors often roll over into our home life. Most of us never think about the fact that we spend the majority of our waking hours in our work environments. The unfortunate part of this is that the majority of us are ill prepared for the job market, often falling into our careers, as opposed to planning them.

Have you ever experienced the humiliation of having an idea you've created get credited to your boss? Your work is too important to give up; however, like everyone else you need a paycheck. Regardless of hang-ups, insecurities, harassment or misunderstandings, the body must perform and the will must survive. The responsibilities you face are similar to the male peers who work beside you and, as always, women's average pay is still equivalent to $.70 for every $1.00 the men earn.

Once you complete the workday, if you have children, you must tend to their needs. You become chauffeur, maid, answering service, cook, provider, referee, organizer, and counselor while providing a shoulder to cry on. Whose shoulder do you use? Who relieves your pressures? Medical studies link unrelieved stress to high blood pressure, ulcers, elevated blood sugar (diabetes), nervous disorders, bowel discomforts and exasperation of herpes.

In spite of all you do, remember, you are still a woman inside, and out. Meditation, whirlpool, massage, quiet lunches, hairdresser appointments, nail and feet pedicures, and light shopping flings are just a start to alleviate the stressors of life.

THE MIND IS A TERRIBLE THING NOT TO HAVE.

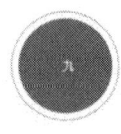

Message from a Serial Killer...

My tall physique and charming wit
Allow women to dream they fit
and once they've fallen for my alluring face
I choke their life spirit into another place

So why am I excited by this
For them it begins as a simple kiss
My hands though strong obscure their fate
Thirteen so far met Heaven's or Hell's gate

Memories stay locked within my brain
Sealed by a father no doubt insane
He burned my skin with a cigarette lit
then locked, no buried, me in a silent pit

For days I hunger, no light in sight
But that was better than dad's tortured fright
Soon light would come and with beer in hand
Dad would beat and kick, well I'll be damned

Why would my mom allow my world?
To stay tormented in a relentless swirl
She desperately inside wanted me to hug
But succumbed always to her cloud of drugs

So here I am released upon
The frail, the meek, the unsuspecting ones
They want to believe all I promise
Why, because think I'm Henry Thomas

A country boy from Texas south
With a polite drawl from my southern mouth
A mask no doubt from the crimes I've done
Worse with time, though they started with one

I didn't mean to lock the door
That janitor was always a boor
The fire was only meant to scare
But spread to quickly, he burned in there

After seeing such a sight
Inside I knew my future plight
Death controlled by my own hands
I then set out to make these plans

Soon I became another face
My soul was dark, destroyed, displaced
Others need drugs to commit their crimes
For me it's a whim and just the right time

One was found in a party place
Another just went to lock her gate
A third needed cigarettes from a local store
And yes there were many, many more

So I strolled along on a sunny day
Blending with those who passed my way
Caught not once for a single crime
Never punished by doing time

This incompetence allows me to escape
And continue in my grueling fate
So let me glance among the crowd
Finding what is not allowed

Then another victim strolled my way
I glanced and knew she was my next prey

> I bought a ticket to where she went
> And took time with my descent
>
> In the crowd we stood, awaiting the train
> She boarded, I stalked, but we walked the same
> Oblivious to her own demise
> But not needed when I collect my prize

CHAPTER NINE
When Women Are Safe & Unsafe

What you know is different than what you think you know, and what you don't know can get you "kilt". That's worse than being killed, because before you get there, you are usually maimed, tormented, disfigured, and tortured. Violence against women takes many forms but extracts the same intolerable suffering.

This chapter will explore the many various facades of abuse against women, some familiar and some not. These include domestic abuse, honor crimes, murder, rape, feticide and female circumcision, and eugenics. In addition to educating women in avoidable ills, we hope to share information on how women can protect themselves against these abuses and learn to "Stay Safe".

Paranoia is not the answer but a few sensible practices can make all the difference in staying protected.

Domestic Abuse:

Domestic abuse is an equal opportunity employer and selects its employees from every race, age, ethnicity, sexual orientation, disability and financial tier. Over 2 million women are abused each year in this country. The physical, mental, financial, sexual and emotional turmoil from the abuse is difficult to conceptualize, especially coming from a loved family member, partner, spouse or friend. Early on, your admirer may seem attentive, generous and protective in ways that later turn out to be frightening, controlling and abusive.

There is always a remorse period called the "honeymoon stage" before the violence like clockwork starts again. Thus, a vicious circle ensues and remains unbroken. Violence tends to increase with drugs, alcohol, monetary woes and pregnancy. Helplessness is shrouded by shame, and few victims seek much needed assistance. Their peril is even more solidified by the fact they do not recognize the abuse, and feel they are the cause and blame.

The abuser has then succeeded, because their main thrust is power, control isolation, and it doesn't stop with you. Your children are also abused in these environments, so take off the blinders and never leave your children alone. If you are in an abusive relationship and truthfully seek help you must realize one important fact, something must change. It won't however, unless you can say yes to the following questions:

1. Am I willing to leave my partner for good?
2. Do I want my children in a better environment?
3. Am I able to become financially capable of taking care of myself and/or my children at some point in time?

4. Can I work on a plan to escape, even though I can't leave right now?

5. Will I refuse to let anyone ever hit me again?
6. Can I be a strong person by myself?

If you can't answer "yes" honestly, you are not ready to stop being a victim of domestic violence, and this is what you have to look forward to in your future:

- Always being afraid of your partner.
- Forced sexual activity, otherwise known as rape.
- Constant unsupported accusations.
- Stalking your every move.
- Imprisoning you in your own home.

Possibly become one of the 2 million injuries and 1,300 deaths that occur each year from domestic violence.

Effects of abuse, such as depression, anxiety, panic attacks, substance abuse and post-traumatic stress disorder.

However, if you are serious about seeking help, many resources are available. Here are a few helpful tips

Develop a plan to escape even if you are not quite ready.

Start packing a suitcase and keep it out of the house, like in a garage, backyard or at a neighbor or friend's house.

Fill it with a change of clothes, toiletries, pajamas, non-perishable packaged snacks, money even if you have to put away a little at a time (especially change), extra house/car keys, pre-paid phone card or disposable cell phone, copies of your children's important papers like immunization/birth certificate records and phone numbers of friends/relatives. You may need these to re-enroll your children in a different school district.

Go to the home of a friend or relative in an emergency.

Visit and gather information from local shelters where you can get support and assistance and ask about rules for children if needed.

Have available phone numbers of the local police and only use them when you are in an emergency or life-threatening situation.

Do not use drugs or alcohol because you need to think clearly.

If you are fortunate enough to escape you may still face social/physical isolation, psychological and economic entrapment, lack of social support, religious and cultural repercussions, fear of social judgment threats, intimidation over custody or separation, immigration status issues, disabilities or lack of viable alternative.

But the public, community, social and healthcare systems can help.... and you and/or your children will be free.

National Organizations
National Domestic Violence Hotline
http://www.ndvh.org
800-799-7233

National Coalition Against Domestic Violence
303-839-1852
www.ncadv.org

National Network to End Domestic Violence
202-543-5566
www.endabuse.org

National Resource Center on Domestic Violence
800-537-223

According to The Centers for Disease Control, in 2003 over $8.3 billion was spent on medical care, mental health services, and lost productivity associated with domestic violence.

Murder Against Women

Sometimes women just don't get it right.

"In 2005, 1,181 women were murdered by an intimate partner. That's an average of three women every day. Of all the women murdered in the U.S., about one-third is killed by an intimate partner". (Bureau of Justice Statistics)

What makes a woman stay with a partner that may, might, or will kill her? Even pregnancy does not protect a woman from her abuser, as homicide is the third leading cause of death for pregnant women. Do we, as a society, provide no way out for these ill-fated victims, or are they responsible for their own fate? Instead of merely reporting these grueling statistics we must give them personalization and meaning. Women who are murdered do not live in a vacuum. They have family, friends, co-workers and associates. The desire to not get involved must be out-weighed by the value of human existence.

Honor Crimes

"Honor crimes." are intended to protect a family, clan or tribal honor by murdering a female family member who is thought to have brought shame from unacceptable behavior. Those committing the "womanicide" believe such actions are supported within religious and ethnic beliefs. Accusations of sexual infidelity, abduction, criminal arrest, or rape provide justification for these killings, often infiltrating into existing formal legal systems. The sequelae of such actions maintain society's male domination and phallic control. The role of women becomes subservient, undermined, exploited, dictated and women become stripped of the right to make any autonomous decisions.

The international human rights law recognizes honor crimes as a form of violence against women, because it violates a women's "right to life and security, freedom from torture and cruel, inhuman, and degrading treatment." International law obligates states to protect women from gender-based violence, including by family members, and to disqualify "honor" as a legal defense for acts of violence against women. Additional support from the Universal Declaration of Human Rights in

Article 5 states; "no one shall be subjected to torture or to cruel, inhuman or degrading treatment or punishment, with equal protection under the law." However, these cultural crimes pre-date modern legalities, deeply embedded in countries like Argentina, Bangladesh, Brazil, Ecuador, Egypt, Guatemala, India, Iran, Jordan, Lebanon, Pakistan, Palestine, Peru, Syria, Turkey, and Venezuela. Here the inalienable rights of everyone are based on gender not humanism.

Even in the United States lesser punishments have been given calling justification for honor crimes mitigating circumstances. In one case a man was sentenced to only four months in prison by a Texas judge for murdering his wife in front of their 10-year-old child for adultery. These crimes are looked at from the perspective of the perpetrator and public supported sympathy has allowed acceptably substituting the term honor crimes for crimes of passion.

Rape:

The need to sexually control someone against his or her will is pathetic.

Rape is about power. Anyone can be a rape victim, regardless of gender or sexual orientation. White men commit most of the rapes in the U.S., yet, if you examine the penal system, more men-of-color are incarcerated. Who is most likely to be a victim? Black women.

A 1991 study performed by the National Victim Center of Arlington, Va., found that within this racial group, one out of every three American women would be raped in her lifetime -- most before they reach age 18. The past acceptable "sexual property" dogma of slavery have left some Black woman victims feeling it's not really rape and their perpetrators burying their crimes in the fallacy that these women are naturally "over sexed".

Women with disabilities are especially victimized, with a 50 percent higher risk of being sexually assaulted. Often powerless and limited by their disability, they are viewed as unable to protect themselves. Rapists find them easy prey with the attitude they should be glad someone wants to rape them.

Even more injurious, women are often blamed for enticing their attacker by solicitous dress and mannerisms and are not deserving of the right to say "no". Instead of being sympathized as a victim, some actually believe "they ask for it". That only shields the perverted behavior associated with a rapist.

Rape is not prejudiced to heterosexual couples or to penetration with a penis

Did you know?
Other women can rape women?
Violence occurs in 1 out of 4 lesbian relationships?
Most of these crimes go unreported

Sexual Violence Statistics
In 2005, victims age 12 or older experienced 191,670 rapes/sexual assaults.

92% of rape or sexual assault victims in 2005 were female.

Crime-statistics indicate that most female rape or sexual assault victims knew their attacker. 38% of women assaulted by a known offender were friends or acquaintances of the rapist, and 28% were intimate partners.

In 2005, only 38.3% of all rapes and sexual assaults were reported to law enforcement.

41% (38, 79 of reported forcible rapes were cleared (usually by arrest) by law enforcement.

Almost a third (30.1%) of all sexual assaults occurred at or in a victim's home.

Characteristics associated with a positive legal outcome in sexual assault cases include being examined within 24 hours of the assault, having been assaulted by a partner or spouse, having been orally assaulted, and having genital trauma.

Rape survivors who had the assistance of an advocate were significantly more likely to have police reports taken and were less likely to be treated negatively by police officers.

Victims of rape are 13 times more likely to develop two or more alcohol-related problems and 26 times more likely to have two or more serious drug abuse-related problems than non-crime victims.

Feticide:

This refers to the deliberate killing of a fetus. In 2004, the Unborn Victims of Violence Act was enacted by Congress and signed by President Bush. It states the unborn fetus is recognized as a victim and if injured or killed during the commission of certain violent crimes, punishable. Unfortunately, other countries have acted with less esteem and feticide is acceptable and female specific. This is more common in those societies where the perception of women and their role in society are diminished, and women are granted less respect and worth. Also sons are considered more profitable and are able to secure work which brings in family income. In countries like China, Afghanistan, Pakistan, Nepal, and South Korea, female feticide is too long considered traditional. The British Medical Journal, Lancet, reports approximately 50 million female fetuses have been victims of feticide in China and another 43 million in India alone. With the access to ultrasounds and their documentation of gender (sometimes wrong), this has placed, especially in wealthy hands, an easier road towards female feticide.

Female Circumcision vs. Genital Mutilation

Female Circumcision

Female circumcision is supported by senseless, yet traditional and deep-rooted beliefs. Everyone seems to be on the cultural bandwagon except often the one being circumcised. This unfortunate ritual has left many female victims maimed, deformed and emotionally traumatized. I have often been saddened when I recount one couple's request to circumcise their newborn daughter. I replied, "What is down there to circumcise?"

Female genital mutilation

This is an unfortunate culturally driven practice that removes the external genitalia, in particular the clitoris and in addition may also stitch close the opening to the vagina. This should not be confused with female circumcision that can have medical practical applications.

Female circumcision

The clitoris, an extremely sensitive area of the female genitalia, and is covered by a "hood" of tissue called the prepuce. Sebaceous glands that lie around the clitoris provide lubrication to the area, but if they do not function properly, the area becomes dry and adhesions can form between the clitoris and prepuce. The clitoris then remains covered, and unable to be stimulated during sexual excitation. This has led to the development of psychosocial illnesses, marital discordance and divorce. Also seen in young children, where bacteria enter and contaminate the area, producing smegma that becomes trapped. Children then complain of irritation, irritability, frequency, and urgency and often scratch or masturbate to achieve relief.

Women can also have too much tissue covering the clitoris, which is called redundancy, and can lead to similar problems. In this simple procedure, female circumcision, only the prepuce, or outer skin covering is cut and the clitoris is exposed. There is usually no bleeding, or at least very little when performed properly. The area is then cleansed of contaminant debris or of smegma that occasionally is formed into stones of various sizes and post-procedure symptoms improve.

Female genital mutilation:

Deliberate removal of the external part of the clitoris partially or totally is called clitoridectomy. This causes loss of sensation in the female genital area and the pleasure associated with intercourse. Since many of these procedures are performed as ritualistic in third world countries, tools used include scissors, razor blades, old rusty knives, or broken bottlenecks. Other methods include prickling the genitals with nettles until they are swollen enough to be charred.

More severe mutilations are called infibulations where the clitoris and labia are sliced off. The vaginal opening is then closed by stitching the raw edges together with thorns, leaving only a pinpoint opening. The girl's legs are tied together for weeks in order to "heal" and tiny branch is inserted to maintain an opening for urination.

Over 2 million involuntary female circumcisions are being performed every year, mainly in African countries with 6,000 daily victims. Up to 1/3 of young girls die from this procedure if no antibiotics are given.

Maintaining such a pinpoint opening enhances male pleasure during intercourse at the expense of excruciating pain to the woman.

This is also one of the theories behind the escalation of HIV/AIDS in Africa, as these young innocent girls were more desirable to foreigners with money looking for sexual gratifications. Also, culturally, an uncircumcised woman was considered dirty, oversexed and unmarriageable; fate women from any country wouldn't want to endure.

Eugenics: Supported Racism or a Historical Disgrace?

Medically sanctioned selective genocide was cloaked in the term "eugenics", popular in the early 1900's and justified to improve the American populations' genetic composition through racial purification.

Sound familiar? Could the eugenic movement in the US have actually fueled Hitler's criminal annihilation of over 6 million Jews? During the war crimes tribunal in Nuremberg after World War II, prominent Nazi leaders cited the US as inspirational for their own mass non-consented sterilization of 450,000 victims over a decade.

Based on popular theories of the time, eugenic philosophy sought justification. Mendelian geneticist believed certain traits were passed to offspring from parents and/or previous generations. In addition, Friedrich Weismann's germ plasma theory identified germ or reproductive cells as the means of transferring these traits. Staunch eugenicists later concluded based on this literature that concerning transferable traits like alcoholism, mental retardation, schizophrenia, bipolar disorder, depression, poor intelligence and undesirable phenotypes (appearances) could be erased from future generations through selective, non-consented sterilization.

In 1912, the First International Congress of Eugenics was held and supported by many prominent individuals. They included President Leonard Darwin, the son of Charles Darwin who formulated the "survival of the fittest" and "evolution" concepts. Also affiliates were Winston Churchill, future Prime Minister of the United Kingdom, Auguste Forel, famous Swiss pathologist and Alexander Graham Bell, American inventor of the telephone. Those who later contributed significant financial boosts were Dr. Clarence Gamble of Procter and Gamble and James Hanes of famous the hosiery company.

Charles Benedict Davenport, the "father of the American eugenics movement", set up in the US, the Eugenics Record Office (ERO), in 1910. Here were collected hundreds of thousands of medical histories from unsuspecting Americans, with selections based on race, intellect, ethnicity, immigration status, and economic or social poverty. The focus was human population improvement via selective breeding.

"We do not want word to go out that we want to exterminate the Negro population," stated Margaret Sanger, American eugenicists. Now sometimes we are accused of taking statements out of context, so here is the entire quote:

"We should hire three or four colored ministers, preferably with social-service backgrounds, and with engaging personalities. The most successful educational approach to the Negro is through a religious appeal. We don't want the word to go out that we want to exterminate the Negro population..."

This was in reference to her founding and institution of the "Negro Project", which was a plan to focus on sterilization of the poor and immigrant, with emphasis on African-Americans. This later transformed into Planned Parenthood, whose initial purpose was to maintain American population integrity by preventing the passage of era accepted undesirable traits.

Sanger aligned herself with the eugenic philosophy and was an invited speaker at Klu Klux Klan rallies.

Starting with Indiana in 1907, eugenic boards were established in 31 states. Often with a minimal number of members, decisions for sterilizations were made with little to no interference and based on anyone's subjective impression of undesirability. Over 60,000 Americans were involuntarily sterilized, with 30,000 in California alone. Most were completely unaware their fertility had been removed. These common practices on the considered "less desirable" lasted until 1963. Some eugenic laws allowing forcible sterilization have stayed on the books until as late as 2003.

Recently, past eugenic behaviors, which targeted area women, mainly African-Americans and the poor, has come to light in North Carolina. With 2,000 sterilization victims still alive in North Carolina, their voices have recently become audible. North Carolina Governor Beverly Perdue, in a NBC interview stated, "You can't rewind a watch or rewrite history. You just have to go forward and that's what we're trying to do in North Carolina." Although the state issued an apology for its involvement in this eugenic behavior, no known financial compensation has been awarded to the victims.

During the "Eugenic Era", anyone could make a recommendation to the state's eugenic board, to rid society of any and all of their preconceived unfavorable humans. One candidate was approved on the simple statement she was, "feeble-minded and promiscuous ... schoolwork was poor and that she does not get along well with others." Initially, non-entitled obstructive passage of traits like mental illness and retardation soon included any racial or ethnic bias and ended with sterilizations based on complaints as simple as," She's too ugly."

Women Protect Yourself

There are many things than women can do to protect themselves against abuses and stay safe. Often victims are targeted by their attitude, mannerisms and compliance. If you are engrossed in conversation on your cell phone, inattentive to your surroundings, you may be victim.

Safety Tips

Always keep your keys out when going to your car. You don't want to be caught fumbling through a cluttered purse for them. Stay off the cell phone until you reach your destination. If you think someone is following you, cross the street. Always trust your instincts.

Dark and desolate parking lots scream "unsafe" and if possible use valet parking, especially in unfamiliar areas.

Medical alert buttons, panic remote key alarms or anything that makes a loud noise are good to have when you are out alone, walking to parking lots or deserted streets.

If legal, keep mace or pepper spray handy at home and on the road.

Invest in a home security system or a dog.

If keeping an extra set of keys outside, invest in a lock box; don't leave it loose under a mat or plant.

Try not to be alone, so take a friend when shopping, eating at a restaurant, going to a movie or a night out on the town. Fashion is one thing but dressing to attract a rapist can be avoided. Take a good look at yourself in the mirror before going out.

Never leave a drink unattended, and if you do, pitch it and order another one.

If traveling bring a simple door wedge to place under your hotel door for added protection and keep the doors double locked when inside.

Take a self-defense or safety orientated class.

Empowerment is the solution to abuse.

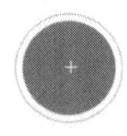

Money seems to go before it comes
But that's just for the lucky ones
For most, it was never there
Despite our purse of plastic ware
Still we spend with unforced hand
A signature, the only demand
Until the monthly bills are due
And we don't have the revenue

CHAPTER TEN
The King is in His Counting House

I was not good at saving money...ever. It was not for the lack of trying, it just wasn't in my genes. Neither were neatness, structure, efficiency or organization and I think those are prerequisites. As life progressed, and I moved through the metamorphic stages of youth to adulthood, the need to know about financial organization was even more important, yet still missing. Upon entering the job market, I worked long hours and soon those demanding and unwavering allegiances, overworked existences and personal exhaustions put even more of a damper on the entropy within my financial life.

Now most of us have that little voice of consciousness you hear in the back of your head that reminds you of things you should and shouldn't do; instead, I had my mother. She was unlike any other. Despite her 5'3 frame, she had firm beliefs and if you crossed her, it could be asphyxiating. However, she had a strong devotion to her family that was admirably insurmountable.

To her credit, my mother had great budgeting skills, a necessity because those around her did not. With limited funds, she proudly maintained a beautiful home for over 30 years, regardless of the myriad of jack-legged contractors, plumbers, electricians and handymen that traversed the premises.

My mom attempted to educate and advise me on my own erratic but American acceptable spending habits, trying to get me to see the importance of saving, paying bills on time, and finding thrifty ways of buying good products. I can still remember her filtering through the numerous clothing racks at Marshalls where out of 50 garments, my mom could find the only one discounted from Saks. However, at the time, I was not teachable. Good thing my daughter was.

Still our financial conversations would always end with her reminding me of the old adage, "Mary saved and Martha didn't."

I told her to make sure they put on my tombstone, "Here lays Martha"

Of course, in writing this chapter I needed some help. I turned to my daughter who majored in finance, and is masterful (thanks sweetie). I asked her the age-old questions, "How do you get your finances on track? Where do you even start?" I need something for people who don't have time to read the volumes of information already out there, just a quick fix. Here was her advice.

First, there is no quick fix. It is going to take time and commitment to change old, established and frivolous spending habits into practical, much appreciated new ones that focus on budgeting and sensible spending.

I. Start with an understanding of where your money goes.

For a week, keep a "spending diary." Track all your purchases from big ticket items to that tiny stick of gum...e-v-e-r-y-t-h-i-n-g! Record date, amount and what you spent it on. Then, take a long look to see where your money is going. Include the unexpected splurges, multiple trips to the ATM and handouts to friends and family members. Once you understand where your money goes, it will be easier to stay responsible in providing necessities, but at the same time, trim the fat.

II. Keep your bills handy.

You can't pay them on time if you don't know where they are. Keep a mail basket (of adequate size to hold a week's mail) handy and when you get the mail, put it there immediately. Take a minute to go through and throw out the junk mail and advertisements, but first tear off your address part and shred it. This helps protect your personal information. If others are also getting the mail, train them to do the same.

III. Prepare a realistic and honest assessment of your finances.

Leaving nothing out. This may take a short trip to an office supply store to stock up on black markers, file folders and storage containers. Make sure you have a folder for every bill due. Once you outline the depth of your financial situation, your files will help translate it into a format easy to understand.

IV. Develop a reasonable financial payment plan.

This should include the payment of all bills based on your accessible income. Essential bills should come first, they are listed below. For all other bills and debts, pay in accordance to its level of importance (which can be assessed by how much of an interest rate you are paying, how much debt is outstanding, prepayment penalties and/or the late payments assessed if late), and call to try and make payment arrangements for the rest. Sometimes paying a little is better than not paying at all. Also pay bills on time (good for your credit score and avoid additional late charges). If you are electronic savvy, take advantage of automatic bill withdrawal payments, but make sure they are still recorded. Some creditors will offer lower interest rates with these types of payments, and you save on the monthly stamp and envelope. It is important to set aside time at least once a week in a quiet room to implement your plan and review your progress.

Now let's get organized!!!

First determine how much income you have to work with. Sit down and make a list of all your income each month. Include everything.

YOUR INCOME

- Salary (after taxes), tips, commission
- Rental property income
- Social security benefits
- Alimony or child support
- Other supplemental income

Ever think about creatively making extra income. Try tutoring, home repair, flower arranging, counseling, baking, teaching a musical instrument, or starting a small business on the side with your talents, for extra income.

Assets

Take a minute to look at your assets. This may be a source of additional monies in an emergency or time of need. List everything you own (not still owe on because that means it is not truly yours!). Include cash, Certificates of Deposits (commonly known as CDs), bonds and investments. You will often need this information for other things like a loan or purchasing a home, but keep it secure.

Now, that's what you have to work with.

Next list all your bills that you have to pay and divide them into the groups listed below.

I. Essential Bills

Basic Monthly Essential Bills: Necessary for existence.

    A. Rent/Mortgage
    B. Telephone (Home and Mobile)
    C. Electric
    D. Gas
    E. Food
    F. Transportation
    G. Other

These are essential monthly bills you must pay to maintain a minimum daily existence. They have to be paid, but there are ways to reduce them.

Rent/Mortgage:

You should not spend more than 25 to 30 percent of income on your rent or mortgage. If you are, look into refinancing your mortgage for lower available interest rates or renegotiate your apartment lease to a lesser amount if it is up for renewal.

Telephone Bills:

According to Nielsen, a market researcher, consumers shell out a little more than $1,300 a year for phone services (roughly $40 a month for a landline and $70 a month for wireless plans).

Landline:

Drop extra charges for services you may not use like call waiting or call forwarding.

Get rid of your landline if you are not using it. In a CBS news report, one in four households with cellular phone service did not have a landline as of May 2010.

Look into measured use service available for a small monthly fee. Shop around, because some services have free incoming calls).

Other alternatives include internet calling, which may be free or low cost, like Skype and Google voice.

Cell Phones:

Shop other carriers for better deals when your contract is up. Even if you have a plan, always check for new deals, pre-pay or no contract phones.
Look for free in-network calling and ask friends and family to join the network.
Make sure your plan matches your talk time.

Skip cell phone insurance. You can pay $7-$10 dollars per month and still another $50.00 to replace what is usually a refurbished phone. However, if you have a very expensive phone, you may want insurance.

Don't get all the extra gadgets if you are not using them.

Don't hold when paying by the minute.

Minimize non-free calls like toll calls or 4-1-1 (use 1-800-GOOG-411 instead, it's free!).

Look into employers, unions, alumni associations and other discount membership groups that offer deals on cell phone services.

Look into bundling if you have multiple services like cable, internet, and phone with one carrier, but be in a position to pay a larger bill when it comes, instead of several smaller ones.

Go unlimited on services you use frequently.

Utility Bills

Next, let's look at utility bills. We should all be looking at ways to save the environment. Invest in energy-saving bulbs around the house, timers or just have everyone conscious enough to turn off the lights when not in use. Remember they have sleep timers on most remotes, so the television does not have to play all night to an invisible viewer. Also utilities can be unexpectedly high depending on the season, with increased use of the air conditioner in the summer, or heat in the winter. Find ways to insulate against drafts from improperly sealed windows or doors, and look into getting on budget bills with your local utility company. That way you have a set amount expected to spend each month. The Environmental Protection Agency's Energy Star program (energystar.gov) offers a free calculator to do a home energy audit and can provide a referral list to a professional in your area.

Food

Get a little more savvy with food expense. Start with planning meals. Make a list when you go grocery shopping and try to stick to it. Also look into coupons. It's not as time consuming as you think, and it's even better when the item is already on sale or when you shop on double coupon days. Get a coupon organizer to make them easier to find. There are a few on-line sites that send you weekly coupons like Krazy Coupon Karen and Coupon Suzy. TheGroceryGame.com can also be helpful. Try to reduce eating out, it is usually more expensive, and remember adding a pet is going to increase your food (and miscellaneous) bill – they may be cute, but they are very expensive.

Organic foods can sometimes be healthier because they claim to use less pesticides, are not genetically modified and animals are not hormonally augmented. However, they can be expensive. If you must do organics, keep them limited to meats, fruits and vegetables. Other staples can come from more traditional and less expensive grocery stores.

Transportation:

If you need to get back or forth to work or school, try to find ways to cut expenses. Car pool to save on gas or get monthly bus or train passes if public transportation is cheaper than driving. Look for gas specials and fill up. The recent economic stimulus package allowed employers to increase the transit benefit they can offer their employees from $120 to $230 a month. Talk with human resources to see if you can deduct this money pre-tax from your paycheck.

Second, list all other monthly non-essential bills and when they are due. See if there is a way to cut them down too.

II. Non-Essential Bills

Non-essential bills are bills that still need to be paid, usually on a monthly basis, but are not essential to survival.

    A. Insurances
       Health
       Dental
       Life

    B. Car Note
    C. Cable Service
    D. Credit Cards
    E. Loans

    F. Other Debt

Variable Expenses

Variable Expenses are expenses that vary, in terms of total amount due, and may not necessarily be paid monthly.

    A. Medical expenses
    B. Personal care
    C. Insurances:
    D. Homeowners/Renters
    E. Car Insurance
    F. Laundry/Dry Cleaning
    G. Clothing
    H. Entertainment

Examine these bills carefully and then start making some phone calls. See where you can cut costs, negotiate interest rates or bundle services. Also cut out what you don't need.

Now that you have an agenda, it's time to develop a financial folder to help organize all your bills.

ORGANIZE FINANCIAL FOLDERS

Make a folder for each expense. Place a divider between those due before the 15th and what is due after. Alphabetize each section. This helps to see what can be paid out of each check. Also on the folder list the bills due dates, to avoid paying them late and accruing additional charges. Inside the folder keep track of statements, payment amount, date of payment with check number, if applicable, and remaining balances. Find out which bills have grace periods, which gives you a period of time by which to pay late without incurring a fee, and document that too.

Now you have to organize any remaining debt into similar folders the only way to get out of debt is list what you owe.

Start making arrangements to make monthly payments, no matter how small; they add up over time. You can also contact your debtors who are, often willing to reduce the bill amount if paying in full.

Subtract bills paid from available income. What you have left can be divided into two parts (70/30). The larger amount should be put into a savings account. The smaller amount is for you, so treat yourself. It doesn't have to be big or expensive. Treat yourself to a nice lunch, manicure or massage. It's money you work for so don't forget yourself.....don't ever forget yourself.

Protect Your Checking Account

A. Make sure you have Overdraft Protection. It is not only criminal to intentionally write a bad check, but you can incur unreasonable fees. Often your bank can link your account to credit card, savings or money market account, which can cover when funds are not sufficient.

B. Be careful when giving out your account number and bank routing information.

C. Always check your statements.
D. Don't leave your blank checkbooks out around the house, all guests are not honest.

E. If you must list a phone number on checks, use a mobile instead of a home phone number. It may make it harder to link the number with your home address. If not needed, don't list your phone number at all.

Credit card tips

A. Try to minimize the use of your credit cards; they should be occasionally, like for trips or emergencies. If there are only a few charges each month, the charges will be easier to verify, which should be done each month, and you will be able to spot fraudulent charges easily.

B. Check your interest rate. Often cards start with a low rate and then raise it later. If this happens, contact the credit card company and if they are not willing to negotiate a lower rate, look for another credit card company with better rates. If there are transaction fees, call to verify what they are for so you can avoid them in the future.

C. Try to consolidate multiple cards into one or two. However, check the balance, transfer interest rates, and one-time fees.

D. Some credit cards have a grace period on purchases, and if you pay your balance in full every month, you can avoid interest charges.

E. Look for debit or credit cards that give you cash back on purchases.

You may need help with paying your credit cards, especially if:

You can't afford to pay the minimum balance on your credit card each month.

Can't seem to pay bills on time, especially after trying.

You are avoiding the creditors and collection agencies that are calling, demanding payment.

If you are having trouble paying your credit card, you may want to contact a debt management company or credit counselor.

Try to avoid debt settlement companies for the reasons outlined below.

Debt Management Companies

- Usually non-profit.
- Free or minimal fees.
- Utilize professional credit counselors.
- Many agencies are also approved through HUD and can also assist with mortgage counseling.

- Work to eliminate balances within five years.
- Work with creditors to negotiate payment arrangements.

Debt Settlement

- Charge fees up to 15% of total balance due.
- Usually for-profit agencies.
- Minimal financial education provided.
- Accounts often fall further behind or end up being written off.
- Negative impact on credit for up to seven to ten years
- Creditors may involve their attorneys and pursue legal proceedings against the customer working with these agencies.

Always ask which type of agency you are working with.

Another option is to call a credit counselor. Below is the contact information of two credit card counselors:

A. The National Foundation for Credit Counseling (www.nfcc.org)   1.800.388.2227)

B. The Association of Independent Consumer Credit Counseling Agencies (www.aicca.org) 1.866.703.8787)

Other Tips

A. Keep all receipts, separate them into a business pile and a personal pile. This will be helpful during tax time. Keep receipts of all bills paid in full.

B. Balance your checkbook. Get duplicate checks to help you keep records.

C. Reduce your number of credit cards. Limit them to no more than 3.

D. Reduce the trips to the ATM and go to the ones associated with your bank to reduce fees. Set up alerts for withdrawals so you can keep track. Go once a week and take out what you need and don't go back. Learn to budget what you have.

E. Keep a small basket to keep mail in when you get it out the mailbox. That keeps important bills handy. Immediately throw away all the junk mail and circulars.

F. Cancel all unused accounts, including bank accounts or credit cards. Write a letter formally closing them or get a statement of closure from the source. This will protect you from future liability if someone else is able to use them after closing them.

G. Try to minimize your bank accounts and keep everything at one bank. It keeps things simple and easy to track.

H. Make a list of all your open Money Markets, Savings, CDs, IRAs and Mutual Funds to see if they can be consolidated too.

I. Shop smart. Look for discounts, sales and use coupons. Use online price comparisons like Bizrate.com, Pricegrabber.com, Shopzilla.com and Smarter.com, especially for big ticket items. Google search coupon codes for online purchases before you buy. Ask retailers if they offer unadvertised specials or are willing to barter - you will be surprised.

J. See if your membership organizations or employment offers group discounts, especially to movies, events, entertainment and phone services. Many times the Human Resource Department offers free or minimal fees for tax services, insurances and counseling.

Now, have thought about your later life and retirement years?

A. First, invest in your health to make sure you will be around. Maintain a healthy weight or loose what you need to get there. Eat healthy and exercise. Get rid of bad habits like smoking and excessive drinking. Always avoid any illicit drug use.

B. Retirement accounts: Do a little investigating. You don't always need the expense of a financial planner immediately. See what you are able to put away by checking with your human resources or surfing the internet for recent tax laws. Maximize what you can. Look into 401K plans at work that often have automatic deductions taken from your pre-tax pay and direct deposited. One recent study showed retirees will now need to save 126% of their ending salary to maintain their standard of living, taking into account medical expenses and inflation.

C. Look into having a will, you don't want the state to decide where you're hard earned money goes, and tax it again.

    D. Try to pay off most bills and avoid making new ones, especially high ticket ones like a new car that is not affordable. If you are living on limited income, practice smart spending.

Tips on Saving

Sign up for Direct Deposit. Have a certain amount automatically withdrawn, placed in a savings account and don't touch it. However, make sure you still receive a payment stub for your records.

Always break a bill when shopping and put that and any other change you have or find in a jar. Hide the jar in a place like the back of a cupboard or the floor of a closet. Do not touch the jar, or the money contained therein, for at least six months, and then use it to open a savings account. When you accumulate enough, get a CD.

Take advantage of "savings clubs" offered at banks for big expenses like vacations and Christmas.

Each week take out what you need from the ATM (use the one associated with your bank to avoid additional fees) or your bank and don't go back.

The most commonly used credit scores are provided by Fair Isaac Corporation and are known as FICO® scores. They can range from 300 (the worst) to 850 (the best)

What makes up your credit score?

    A. 35% payment history
    B. 30% debt
    C. 10% length of credit history
    D. 10% types of credit used

E. 10% new credit

Repair Your Credit

A. Run your credit report and get the facts. It really is painless. Three main companies track consumer debt and assign credit rating scores. Get copies of your credit reports from all three. You're entitled to a free copy from each bureau every year, and another if you've been turned down for credit.

B. Make sure there are not any erroneous reports. If so, you can write the credit bureau disputing it, and ask for an investigation. If it cannot be supported in 30 days, the information has to be removed, until it is reported. Keep any supporting documents for your claim.

C. Make sure all your personal information is correct.
D. Make sure past credit accounts that were closed are not still listed as open.

Credit Report Companies

Equifax Information Services, LLC
P.O Box 740241
Atlanta, GA 30374
www.equifax.com

1-800-685-1111 (order credit report)
1-888-766-0008 (report fraud)

Experian
P.O. Box 2104
Allen, TX 75013-2104
www.experian.com
1-888-397-3742 (order credit report by phone or report fraud)
1-888-397-3742 (request a copy of report by mail)

Trans Union Corporation
Consumer Disclosure Center
P.O. Box 1000
Chester, PA 19022
www.tuc.com

1-800-888-4213 (to order credit report)
1-800-916-8800 (speak with customer service representative)

Before sending any personal correspondence, check their individual website to make sure the above contact information is current.

Realize how important your credit scores are. You need a good score to buy a home, get a loan for school and sometimes just to get a job. Bad scores will either result in you getting turned down or you will pay much higher interest rates on loans or credit cards. Don't lend what you NEED to get back or co-sign for a loan, especially to family and friends. Pass this advice to your children, because even if you messed up your credit, you can use that information to get them on a good road.

Fraud Protection:

Do not throw out any papers that have your sensitive information like your name, address, and/or social security number. Shred it instead.

Throw away nuisance magazines and advertisements you get in the mail.

Look into fraud protection companies, but don't pay any unreasonable fees. Look for free trials so you can check them out first.

Dedicated to My Friends

I have had the blessed opportunity to listen and be entrusted with the personal health experiences of many special patients, family and friends. This has served as a foundation not only for my professional growth, but for the establishment of long-lasting personal friendships and memorable experiences.

#1

I had my first child at 40 years old, a nightmare for some, but for me, it was the best day of my life. I didn't have to worry about exercising, losing weight, eating right…because at my age you were trying to do those things anyway. The only difference is we usually fail, but I had motivation, that precious soul that was growing in my body. Now four years later I sat in the examining room at the doctor's office, thinking about the many joys my daughter, Jamara and I shared. I thought about last Sunday. Jamara had turned four and I really went all out. "Proud of myself," I thought with a silent smile.

How quickly that smile disappeared, once the doctor began to speak. The words had barely rolled off of his tongue when I found myself in hell. "You have multiple sclerosis," he said.

Not me, I have a little girl who needs me. All of a sudden problems that previously existed in my life were not problems at all. Bad relationships, not enough money, job pressures, too tired, all took a backseat to the news that I would die. Multiple sclerosis is a disease in which your own body begins to attack itself and damages the protective coverings around the cells that make up your brain and spinal cord. The result: slurred speech, muscle weakness, loss of vision, spasms in the arms and legs. Eventually wheelchair bound loss of bowel and bladder functions and death. Not me, I have a little girl who needs me.

With tears flowing inside, I began to make plans. I may not be here for my child but I am going to leave her with as much as I can. It was tough because each day I became sicker and sicker. First I made a list of family members I could entrust with Jamara's care. Then I set out to make a will, and list all my worldly possessions, so my child could go on to college and be somebody, even if I was not there .Next I didn't want her to forget me, forget what I looked like or forget I loved her. I started to make videos of myself talking to her, giving advice, warning her about boys, often stopping for a few moments so my tears would not show on camera.

Some days were better than others. I quit my job, one I loved and worked hard to be promoted chief administrator of my office, but time was limited and Jamara was more important. I spent hours watching her smile, running in the park and occasionally looking back, happy I was watching her.

Months had passed. I was barely able to get out of bed. I tried to stay on the medication but it wasn't working. I took the little pill bottle from my night stand. Empty. What's the use? I rolled over and went back to sleep.

The next morning I felt great. I didn't get my medication filled, and a week later I was feeling like my old self. One minute I was planning a funeral and when I stopped taking the medication I was better. It's not supposed to work like that. I made an appointment to see the doctor, and when I arrived, I found out my regular doctor was on vacation. Instead, I was seen by another doctor. He was kind with a great bedside manner, so I was comfortable telling him my dilemma. Why am I no longer sick? After a few moments he took my hand. "I'm sorry. It was the medication that was making you sick. He said. "I reviewed your chart thoroughly and there has been a mistake. The doctor misread your test and you do not have Multiple Sclerosis." "In fact, you are perfectly healthy."

#2

I had a patient who I came to take care of quite unexpectedly. She was a puritan descendant who really did not like doctors. This patient taught at a small non-traditional Quaker- type school in rural Illinois. She received prenatal care with a midwife and was carrying twins.

When I came to work that morning I was asked to see the patient. She had broken her bag of water around one of the twins, and the doctor on call wanted to abort both babies. Angrily upset, she refused to see that doctor anymore, so I was asked to intervene.

Medicine is also about listening and understanding, so before I gave my opinion I did just that, listened. The patient knew if she aborted both babies, neither would survive. They were only 18 weeks. She wanted to know her risks and did she have any other options. Unfortunately, the best management would be to follow the first doctor's advice. But what about the other twin? Their bag was intact. We talked what might happen if we did nothing. She could go into labor and still deliver both twins prematurely. One twin could deliver and the other could have a delayed-interval delivery, where we could intervene and try to keep that twin inside longer to gain more maturity. Because the bag of water around the one twin was broken, infection could set in that would not only hurt the pregnancy but also the mother. If there is no or insufficient water around the baby with the bag broken, they could develop breathing problems, limb or facial deformities. This was a lot to deal with but the mother was appreciative of options.

She chose to continue the pregnancy, accepting all risk. We tried to keep her in the hospital, but she wanted to go home. She left with instructions to return if any signs of infection and bed rest. The patient was very co-operative and we talked weekly. At about 24 weeks, she called complaining of some pressure, so we asked her to return immediately. She stayed in the hospital for three days, showed no signs of labor or contractions, and some water was re-accumulating around the twin who broke their bag. Things looked promising. Again, she wanted to go home. She felt better and the pressure was gone. I told her I wanted to put in a vaginal speculum to just try and look at her cervix. I could not check her digitally with my fingers because of the baby's bag of water being broken and I did not want to increase her risk of infection. When I was putting the speculum in, I could see the leg of one of the babies. We took her to surgery for an emergency Cesarean Section.

Both babies initially survived. Unfortunately the twin with the bag of water broken had repeated lung problems and eventually dies within a couple years. I saw the mother at a hospital event a couple years later with the remaining twin who was doing well without any problems. She was happy with her decision and said if she had done what the doctors originally wanted her to do, she would have lost both twins. At least she was able to have some time with both.

#3

During my residency, I had the opportunity to meet the "Pasta Lady". We called her that because she owned a small restaurant in town and made fresh pasta. Her linguine…Mamma Mia. She was a typical, middle aged Italian, always full of joy. She came to see us because of feeling full all the time, especially in her lower abdomen. After several tests, we found a large, suspicious-looking mass on her ovary. With heavy hearts, we told this wonderful woman she may have ovarian cancer. "So what's next,' she said. Now comes the hard part. Wanting to cure someone from a dreaded disease, but your hands is partially tied, because no matter how good a doctor you are, the finality is in someone else's hands.

We began to explain the surgery and then the chemotherapy, "You may have nausea, vomiting, lose your hair, not be able to eat...." She stopped us abruptly. "I can't do that, I have to make the pasta." Grateful for our advice but she refused all treatments, knowing she may only have months to live. She said she would continue living her life happy, and when her time came, she would be ready. After that the "Pasta Lady" walked out the door.

Several years passed. I was in my final year of residency and thinking of my future. I wandered into the clinic one early morning and began to do paperwork. Soon others filtered in, and we were chatting while waiting for the patients to be put in the rooms. All of a sudden there was the most delicious smell. It was the aroma of freshly baked pasta, and coming down the hall was the "Pasta Lady". She greeted us all with that jolly smile and said she had come to see us today and brought us lunch. After a thorough exam and ultrasounds, the ovarian mass was gone and both her ovaries looked completely normal. When asked why she came back, the Pasta Lady replied, "I never died."

#4

Next time someone asks if you want to have a hysterectomy, just say no, especially if you are only 25. I now live with a colostomy bag. Here is my story.

My cycles were a little irregular. I wasn't too worried at first, but it was starting to get annoying, having to wear a pad all the time. I never knew when I was going to start spotting. Okay, time to visit the doctor.

He seemed nice, lots of diplomas and awards on the wall. I thought I was in good hands. "You have fibroids" the doctor said. 'We're just going to take out your uterus and everything will be fine. Since we're leaving your ovaries, you won't miss it." Then he added, "It's only for making babies anyway."

I was a little annoyed at his last remark, but since I already had three children, I thought it was okay. After the surgery I did not feel well. Okay, it was just the first day. It's normal. That was what all the nurses were telling me. Now it's day #2 after my surgery and I feel worse. My doctor came around. He was always smiling but not listening. He kept saying I was fine and could be discharged in the morning. The next morning I was throwing up..... everything. I couldn't even keep down water. The nurses called me lazy, I just needed to get up and walk around. The doctor said my insurance wouldn't pay. I was sent home.

Soon the fever and chills set in. I still couldn't eat. My kids helped each other get dressed for school, and I couldn't even say good-bye. Days passed and I stayed in my room, sweat-soaked and sick, I would have frightened Freddy Krueger.

My mother came to check on me. Now it was a week after my surgery. She took me to the emergency room. I was immediately admitted and taken back to the operating room. The doctor's watch had fallen off during my previous surgery, lodged into my bowels, and caused a severe infection. They had to remove a large part of my bowel and now I wear a permanent colostomy bag.

This patient was the secretary at a job I had in an inner city clinic. She asked me to look at her ultrasound report taken before her surgery. There was a small fibroid, not 2 cm. (less than 1 inch) present. She didn't need the surgery. When I asked what was the hardest thing to deal with now, she replied, "Explaining during sex why I have a colostomy bag."

#5

It was the 80's and a different time for newborn survival. I had a patient who broke her bag of water at 23 weeks pregnant, and at the time, no efforts to save premature babies were performed before 28 weeks. My patient was devastated and we cried together. I remember staying up with her all night at the hospital. As her labor progressed and pains became stronger, it was inevitable a little one too early to survive was going to be born.

I notified the newborn nursery, and asked if they would admit the baby, not to try any heroic measures, just for comfort care. Let's at least keep her warm, until it's out of our hands. The director of the nursery was a bullish male, unaccustomed to female professionals, who at the time were few. He refused to take the newborn into the nursery and stated, "When the baby delivers, put it in a pan and cover it with a towel, it will soon die." So I did. I can still see myself, meticulously laying a towel on the inside of the pan, and laying that angelic soul so gently upon it. Then I covered the body, said a prayer and placed the pan in a back room. It was 3:00 a.m.

An hour later I returned to pronounce the baby dead and have it taken to the morgue. Amazingly, the baby was still breathing and had kicked a small part of the towel off the pan. . Just enough to uncover a small area. I called the nursery director again and asked if the baby could be placed in the nursery because she was still breathing. I did not think she would survive, but I could not take her laying and dying in that cold pan, in a back room, alone. Harshly, I was told no. I covered the pan again, said another prayer and waited.

Another hour passed and I went into the back room. The baby had kicked a small part of the towel away from the pan and was still breathing. I called the director of the nursery to have the baby admitted, just for comfort care and once more was told no. I checked on that baby every hour, each time the cover was partially removed and the baby was still breathing. Yet again, each time the nursery director was called, he continued to say no and each time more angrily. I felt it was not admitting this poor baby for comfort care but that I as a woman was challenging his authority. Finally around 8am I called the hospital administrator. This baby had now been lying in a pan for 5 hours, being treated like trash, not the precious life she was, no matter how short-lived. He overruled the nursery director and had the baby admitted to the nursery. Of course they were angry and did nothing but place the baby in a warmer. That's all I wanted anyway. But despite the insurmountable odds of survival, that little girl kept breathing.

I continued to see her mother for annual GYN exams, and to my delight she always brought her daughter. She was like any other little girl, and the way she wanted to play everything in my office, definitely nothing wrong with her. Soon after that I left Atlantic City.

Now I reside in Chicago. I worked at a community hospital on the north side. At the time I did OB ultrasounds in the radiology department. One day as I came to work, I heard someone call my name, "Dr. White". It was an older woman about forty and a teenage girl. I didn't recognize her at first. She then continued, "Remember me. I was your patient in Atlantic City; the one who had the premature baby they said would not survive." She turned and looked at the teenager beside her. That was the little girl I had so gently covered up with a towel, now an honor student at Roosevelt University.

#6

I had started my first office in 1980 in a little town that. It had become infamous because of a bank scandal that involved a high ranking official. At the time, many in the area had lost their money at the bank, so I was paid with fresh eggs, milk, meats and vegetables. It was the best I've ever eaten. I remember one day having a charming middle-aged woman come in. She was neatly dressed with a striking lapel pin. Somewhat embarrassed she began to speak of a vaginal issue. After a gentle exam and a few kind words a smile came over her face. I thought at first my warmth and charm had made her comfortable, or maybe she was just glad the exam was over. I wrote a prescription for Monistat vaginal suppositories (not available over the counter at the time), and had her come back in two weeks.

On her return visit I could smell fresh apple pie as she came through the door. My staff was delighted and so was I. She expressed how happy she was that the medicine worked and her vaginal problems were all gone. 'There's only one thing" she said as she left the office. 'Taste terrible!"

#7

Let me tell you the story of Mr. Gaither.

Even though you choose a medical specialty, you have to rotate through other services. I was doing a rotation in Internal Medicine and I did rounds every morning at 6:00 a.m. with another resident, Mark. Neither of us was interested in Internal Medicine. I wanted to become an Ob/Gyn and he wanted to be a Psychiatrist. Nevertheless, here we are at 6:00 am.

It seemed Mark always had the patients that lingered on forever with multiple medical problems. I, on the other hand, would get the patients who would die shortly after arriving on the floor. One morning while we were writing our notes at the nurses' station, Mark was notified one of his patients, Mr. Gaither had just died. He had oat cell carcinoma of the lungs. I teased Mark because his patients never died. They asked Mark to go to the room and check Mr. Gaither. Once he was pronounced dead, the body could be taken to the morgue.

Mark returned to the desk. He said, 'No pulse, no heart rate, no breathing, I think he's dead." We both began to finish writing on the patient's charts when the elevator opened. Two orderlies passed the desk, pushing a long white stretcher, and headed towards Mr. Gaither's room. Within minutes, they came from the room, with Mr. Gaither's body covered with a white sheet. Just like T.V., only this wasn't television. It was real and sadness came over all of us as they passed the front desk and headed towards the elevator. However, that was short lived because all of a sudden Mr. Gaither sat up.

He was talking deliriously and tears were streaming down his face. We could only make out some of what he was saying, but he kept repeating, "Go back, go back."

Later Mark and I went to Mr. Gaithers room to check on him. He was calmer now, almost peaceful. We asked what happened and this is what he said.

I was at a bridge and on the other side I could see many of my family members who have passed away. As I looked towards them, there was a very bright light. I started on the bridge and could feel the warmth. I wanted to go over there with them, but they kept saying, "Go back, go back." Then I woke up.

Several days later, Mr. Gaither died.

#8

A little knowledge is dangerous.

One day a Spanish lady about 30 years old came to my office. She looked 8 months pregnant. After taking her to one of the examining rooms, I asked my nurse to gather some pregnancy information for her after the visit, and I came into the room. "Good morning", I said cheerfully. After introducing myself I asked, "How can I help you today." She replied in a thick Spanish accent, "You gotta help me doctor, I got a tumor in my belly." Somewhat puzzled I asked why she thought that. "Look at me honey, my stomach is getting big", the patient replied. "You gotta help me.

Still somewhat puzzled, I told the patient she might be pregnant. Immediately she jumped off the table, did a little dance and said, "Oh no honey, I not pregnant. I got my tubes tied and I been partying."

Two months later she delivered a beautiful baby boy. Oh no honey!

Appendix

Annual Screening Guidelines 2011
American College of Ob/Gyn (ACOG)
Routine Well-Woman Gyn Exams

These guidelines include routine screenings, laboratory tests, and immunizations for the annual Gyn exam of non-pregnant women.

I. Annual Gyn Exam

Gyn health evaluation should begin at age 13, and does not need to include a Pap test. This provides an opportunity to detect any Gyn-related problems, discuss menstrual issues, prevention of sexually transmitted diseases, birth control options and body issues that develop when entering adolescence. This evaluation can be individualized to the teen's specific needs and parental comfort,

The annual Gyn exam, regardless of age, should inquire about any current health issues, nutrition, physical activity, sexual behavior, and use of tobacco, alcohol, and drugs.

This exam should include measurements of height, weight, body mass index, and blood pressure.

Starting at 19, the annual exam should include breast and abdominal examinations. It would be helpful to teach and provide information on the self-breast exam.

II. Vaccination/Immunizations

Periodic

Ages 13-18 Years:
Tdap (Tetanus, Diptheria, Pertussis): Once between ages 11-18

years
Hepatitis B vaccine (one series for those not previously immunized)
Human papillomavirus vaccine (one series for those not previously immunized, ages 9-26 years)

Influenza vaccine (annually) Measles-mumps-rubella vaccine (for those not previously immunized)

Meningococcal conjugate vaccine (1 dose at age 13-18 years if not previously vaccinated. Persons who received their first dose at age 13-15 years should receive a booster dose at age 16-18 years)

Varicella vaccine (one series for those without evidence of immunity)

Hepatitis A vaccine
Pneumococcal vaccine

Ages 19-39 Years:
Substitute one-time dose of Tdap for Td booster; then boost with Td every 10 years)
Human papillomavirus vaccine (one series for those aged 26 years or younger and not previously immunized)

Influenza vaccine (annually)
Measles-mumps-rubella vaccine (for those not previously immunized)
Varicella vaccine (one series for those without evidence of immunity)

Ages 40-64 Years: Periodic
Substitute one-time dose of Tdap for Td booster; then boost with Td every 10 years)
Herpes zoster (single dose in adults aged 60 years or older)
Influenza vaccine (annually)

Measles-mumps-rubella vaccine (for those ages 40-54 not previously immunized)
Varicella vaccine (one series for those without evidence of immunity)

Ages 65 Years and Older:
Herpes zoster (single dose, if not previously immunized)
Influenza vaccine (annually)
Pneumococcal vaccine (once)
Td or Tdap every 10 years
Individuals who have or who anticipate having close contact with an infant less than 12 months of age and who previously have not received Tdap should receive a single dose of Tdap to protect against pertussis and reduce the chance of transmission.

6) Varicella vaccine (one series for those without evidence of immunity)

III. Cultures

Sexually active teens and women up to age 25 years should have annual testing for Chlamydia and gonorrhea

From age 19-64, all sexually active women should be tested for HIV infection.

IV. Mammogram

Women should have their first mammogram at age 40, and yearly beginning at 50.

Depending on risk and family history, a baseline mammogram may be suggested before age 40.

V. Risk Factors and Interventions

Bone mineral density screening:

Postmenopausal women younger than age 65, history of a previous fracture as an adult, family history of osteoporosis, Caucasian, dementia, poor nutrition, smoking, thin, low body mass index, estrogen deficiency, poor lifelong calcium intake, alcoholism, poor eyesight, history of falls, decreased physical activity. Certain medical conditions and drugs can be associated with an increase the risk for osteoporosis (softening or loss of bone) and can include

Steroids, thyroid medications, antacids that contain aluminum, proton-pump inhibitors to reduce gastric acid and heart burn, certain antibiotics, seizure medications, water pills, blood thinners, lithium, chemotherapy,

Rheumatoid arthritis, Systemic Lupus Erthematoses, Celiac and Inflammatory Bowel, weight loss surgery, Diabetes, Hyperparathyroidism, Hyperthyroidism, irregular menstrual cycles, low testosterone, Sickle Cell Disease. Leukemia, Lymphoma, breast cancer, depression, Multiple myeloma, Eating disorders, Organ transplants, HIV/AIDS, emphysema, chronic kidney diseases, severe liver diseases.)

Basic guidelines suggest starting colorectal cancer screening at age 50 and continue every 10 years. It may be performed sooner if there is a family or personal history of colorectal cancer, polyps, inflammatory-type bowel disease, chronic ulcerative colitis, or Crohn's disease.

The Td (Tetanus-Diphtheria) or Tdap (Tetanus-Diptheria-Pertussis) vaccine may be recommended if in close contact with an infant younger than 12 months or are healthcare providers. Tdap may be given before conceiving and some institutions are giving after delivery.

Checking Fasting Blood Glucose Testing if overweight, first-degree relative with diabetes mellitus, poor physical activity, high-risk race or ethnicity (Type II Diabetes higher risk if

Latinos, American Indians, Asian Americans and non-Hispanic blacks), history of gestational diabetes mellitus or delivery of a high-birth-weight infant, hypertension, lipid disorders, history of impaired glucose tolerance or impaired fasting glucose level, polycystic ovary syndrome, history of vascular disease, and other clinical conditions associated with insulin resistance.

Fluoride supplementation: Live in an area where there is inadequate fluoride in the water.

Genetic testing/counseling: Considering pregnancy and patient, partner, or family member has a history of genetic disorder or birth defect. History of exposure to teratogens that can cause birth defects (some include Thalidomide, alcohol, tetracycline, radiation, infections like rubella, syphilis, CMV and herpes).

Testing for Anemia or Low Hemoglobin Disorders: Those of Caribbean, Latin American, Asian, Mediterranean, or African descent; History of heavy menstrual bleeding; hepatitis A virus vaccination, chronic liver disease, clotting factor disorders, use of illegal drugs.

Hepatitis B virus vaccination: Patients undergoing hemodialysis, those using clotting factor concentrates, healthcare workers or students with exposure to blood in the workplace or school sites, use of injection (IV) drugs, multiple sexual partners, and history of sexually transmitted diseases.

Hepatitis C virus testing: History of using illegal injection drugs, those receiving clotting factor concentrates before 1987, long-term hemodialysis, persistently abnormal alanine aminotransferase levels, recipients of blood from donors who later tested positive for hepatitis C virus infection and multiple sexual partners.

HIV testing: If there is more than 1 sexual partner since most recent HIV test, a sexual partner with more than 1 sexual partner since most recent HIV test, positive sexually transmitted disease in the past year, IV drug use or invasive cervical cancer. HIV testing should be recommended to women seeking preconception evaluation. Also suggested during prenatal care.

Obstet Gynecol. 2011;117:1008-1015.

VI. Pap smear recommendations: (ASCCP 2006)

Start Pap test at age 21 or three years after becoming sexually active.

Women aged 21 to 30 years should be screened every 2 years using either the standard Pap test or liquid-based cytology.

Women 30 years and older who have had three consecutive normal Pap test can be screened once every 3 years with either screening test.

Women older than 30 years can also be screened with a combination of the Pap test and HPV test. If the results are negative for both tests, they do not need to be rescreened for at least 3 years.

Women aged 65 to 70 years who have had at least three normal Pap tests and no abnormal Pap tests in the last 10 years may stop having Pap tests.

6) Women who have had a hysterectomy (both uterus and cervix removed) do not need to have a Pap test if the surgery was done for a non-cancerous reason.

Women with certain risk factors may need more frequent screening, like those with HIV, immunosuppressed, exposed to diethylstilbestrol before birth, and those with abnormal Pap test.

These are just guidelines, discuss with your health care provider your best options and screening guidelines.

If you don't need a Pap, do not skip your annual Gyn evaluation.

***

Committee Opinion #483, "Primary and Preventive Care: Periodic Assessments," Journal of Obstetrics & Gynecology, 2011.

Standard components of the annual ob-gyn exam

A. Address current health status, nutrition, physical activity, sexual practices, and tobacco, alcohol, and drug use.

B. Physical exam should include height, weight, body mass index (BMI), and blood pressure.
C. Start annual breast and abdominal exams at age 19.
D. Routine annual pelvic exams start at age 21.
E. Test for chlamydia and gonorrhea in all sexually active adolescents and young women up to age 25.

F. HIV testing for all sexually active adolescents and women from age 19 until age 64.

Guidelines for Screening Test for Women by Age

These are a few of the recommendations for patients who do not have risk factors; more frequent and/or other testing may be needed depending on health status; always consult your physician.

Ages 18-39

Blood pressure test
Start at age 21, then every 1-2 years if normal. (<120/80)
If blood pressure between 120/80 and 139/89, check every year
If blood pressure 140/90 or higher discuss with physician.

Breast Self-Exams
Start at age 20 then monthly with annual exam by health provider (after instruction)

Cervical cancer screening
Get a Pap test every 3 years if you are 21 or older.
30 or older, Pap test and HPV test together every 5 years or Pap test
alone every 3 years. There should be 3 consecutive normal Pap test.

Chlamydia test
Test for Chlamydia each year if sexually active.

Gonorrhea test
Test for Gonorrhea each year if sexually active.

HIV test
Anyone at risk including sexually active, drug use or sharing needles should be tested. All women All women ages 13-64 should be offered the test.

Diabetes screening
Get screened for diabetes if blood pressure is > 135/80 or if you take high blood pressure medicine.

Cholesterol test
Start at age 20, and repeat every 5 years.

Thyroid test
Start at age 35 then every 5 years.

Ages 40-49

Blood pressure
Check every 1- 2 years if normal blood pressure. (<120/80)
Check each year if blood pressure between 120/80 and 139/89.
If blood pressure is 140/90 or higher discuss with physician.

Self-Breast exam
Every month with yearly exams by health provider.

Mammogram
Start at age 40 then repeats every year.

Pap test
Pap test and HPV test together every 5 years or Pap test alone every 3 years. There should be 3 consecutive normal Pap test.

Diabetes Screening
Start at age 45 then every 3 years.

Cholesterol test
At age 45, have done every 3 years.

Thyroid test
Every 5 years.

EKG
Start at age 40.

Stress Test
Baseline at age 40.

Ages 50-64

General Health Exam
Every year.

Blood pressure check
Check every 1- 2 years if normal blood pressure. (<120/80)

Check each year if blood pressure between 120/80 and 139/89. If blood pressure 140/90 or higher discuss with physician.

Cholesterol screening
Every 1-2 years.

Screening Colonoscopy
Start at age 50 then every 10 years.

Varicella Zoster Vaccine
For women ages 60and older. Single vaccination; no revaccination

(For Shingles)
required.

EKG
Every 1-2 years.

Self-Breast exam
Every month with yearly exams by health provider.

Mammogram
Every year.

Thyroid test
Every 5 years.

Ages 65 and older

General health Exam
Every year.

Blood pressure check
Check every 1- 2 years if normal blood pressure. <120/80
Check each year if blood pressure between 120/80 and 139/89.
If blood pressure 140/90 or higher discuss with physician.

Mammogram
Every year.

Cholesterol screening
Every 1-2 years.

EKG
Every 1-2 years.

Colonoscopy
Every 5-10 years.

DXA (bone-density testing)
Baseline at age 65 then interval testing based on results

Pneumococcal Vaccine (for Pneumonia)
Single vaccine at age 65

Other

Diabetes
screen every 3 years with BMI>25

Human Papilloma Virus (HPV) Vaccine (Gardasil® and Cervarix®):
For all females between ages 11 and 26. One series of 3 vaccines.

Consider flu vaccine each year during flu season, especially if risk factors: asthma, bronchitis, and smoking

Testing for sexually transmitted infections should be done annually for any woman sexually active.

http://my.clevelandclinic.org/Documents/Family_Health_Centers/womens-health-guidelines.pdf

About the Authors

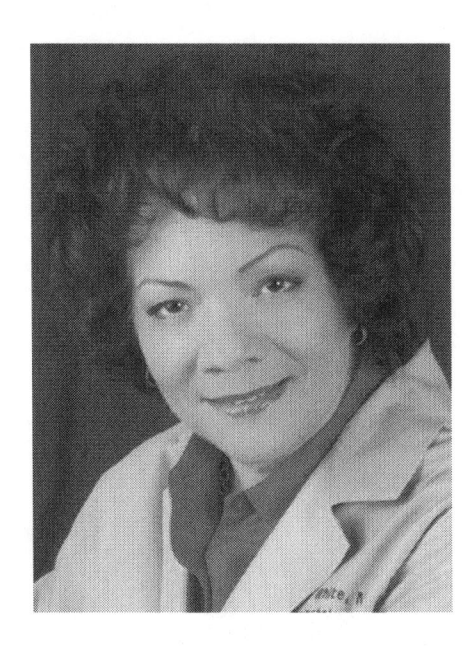

La Lura White M.D. is a dedicated Obstetrician/Gynecologist and Maternal Fetal Medicine Specialist, with over 25 years of personal and professional experience in providing quality health care services to women.

With rising health care cost, personal time restrictions and limited access to medical care, Dr. White realized that it was imperative to empower women with the ability to take a more forward role not only in their own lives, but greatly affect the well-being of their partners, children as well as creating a significant impact on today's work force.

She also realizes the importance of combining nutrition, education, prevention and exercise, with well-developed personal health programs, in order for women to achieve a complete, healthy lifestyle.

Second Opinion 2 is dedicated to assisting women to understand their personal health care needs. Only you can make the decisions that will keep you healthy, and Second Opinion 2 is here to help guide you towards a healthier lifestyle. Let us put our years of dedication and experience to work for you.

It's like always having your doctor with you.

Please visit us on the web at www.secondopinion2.com.

Contact us: info@secondopinion2.com

Pamela D. Burns was an educator, teaching in the Chicago Public School system. Her last employment was at A.N. Pritzker Elementary School, where she was a true inspiration to her students. The Pamela Burns Educational Legacy Fund has been established in her honor.

Ms. Burns spent 22 years working in corporate America prior to transitioning into elementary education.

Ms. Burns always had a remarkable ability to comprehend and present information to others. Her communication skills and desire to help others understand complex issues allowed her to achieve success in all that she has attempted.

Her love of language and writing reached an apex when Dr. White approached her to help put together a book to improve women's understanding of their health care needs. This book is the result of our collaboration.

Ms. Burns graduated from Southern Illinois University with a Bachelor of Science degree in Journalism. She completed her Masters of Arts in Teaching at National-Louis University in Chicago.

On Saturday, January 17, 2009, Ms Burns was laid to rest following a tragic loss. Ms. Burns was not only an amazing person but a professional confidant, AKA sorority sister and dear friend for over 30 years.

In Memoriam

Pamela,

A soul sister and friend

Dear Pam

First I know
You wouldn't want this ...attention
So give me a minute
And I'll be quick

You were my friend
Things were understood
No words needed
But just ask and you would

Ferragamos, if you knew Pam
You knew they were specially made
And when she couldn't decide what color
She bought one in every shade

She had so many first
Her family, her kids, her friends
You couldn't break her
But if she saw you put forth effort
You might get her to bend

So teach the kids in heaven, Pam
Someone special crossed their doors
They took away a gift from us
But children there will learn so much more

Bibliography

Chapter Two, Improving Your Face
1. http://www.fine-skin-care-products.com/facial_toners.html
2. http://www.flawlesscomplexion.com/cleansers.html
3. http://www.natural-skin-care-info.com/natural_skin_care_moisturizer.html

Chapter Three, Au Natural
1. http://www.buzzle.com/articles/interesting-facts-about-cleopatra.html
2. http://www.total-beauty-secrets.com/Egyptian-beauty-secrets.html
3. http://www.total-beauty-secrets.com/Egyptian-beauty-secrets.html
4. http://naturalbeautycare2.blogspot.com/2009/02/ancient-indian-beauty-secrets-with.htm
5. http://www.beautycarehub.com/beauty-secrets/ancient-beauty-secrets.html
6. http://beauty-for-women.com/2011/free-indian-ancient-beauty-tips/

Chapter Four, Not In the Gym Exercises
1. http://www.smartnow.com
2. http://www.fromwith.in/2009/07/16/instant-energy-how-to-breathe-properly/
3. http://www.abc-of-yoga.com/yogapractice/postures.asp
4. http://www.active.com/mindandbody/articles/4-Yoga-Poses-to-Boost-Your-Energy.htm
5. http://www.wikihow.com/Exercise-Your-Eyes

6.http://www.livestrong.com/article/113727-chest-exercises-home-women/#ixzz1iuvG17Ny
7.http://www.fitnessmagazine.com/workout
8.Family Circle July 2006

Chapter Five - Healthy Eating
1.http://www.webmd.com/diet/features/5-foods-fight-hunger-pains
2.http://www.fitday.com/fitness-articles/nutrition/vitamins-minerals/4-zinc-rich-foods-for-healthy-living.html#b

3.http://www.juicing-for-health.com/health-benefits-of-celery.html">http://www.juicing-for-health.com/health-benefits-of-celery.html

4.http://recipes.howstuffworks.com/
5.http://www.essortment.com/aromatherapy-energy-15995.html

Chapter Six - Dietary Changes for Common Health Problems
1.http://www.ithyroid.com/goitrogens.htm
2.http://www.livestrong.com/article/162621-the-best-foods-for-lupus/
3.http://lupus.about.com/od/livingwithlupus/a/LupDiet.htm
4.http://www.ehow.com/way_5412522_diet-lupus.html
5.http://www.livestrong.com/article/14157-breast-cancer-and-diet/#ixzz2E7Qbr3hf
6.http://EzineArticles.com/284849
7.http://ezinearticles.com/?The-Ideal-Diet-for-Hypothyroidism&id
8.http://www.webmd.com/heart-disease/guide/heart-healthy-diet

9. http://www.healthdiaries.com/eatthis/10-health-benefits-of-apples.html
10. http://www.mayoclinic.com/health/diabetes-diet/DA00027
11. http://www.healthaliciousness.com/articles/foods-high-in-calcium.php
12. http://www.healthaliciousness.com/articles/what-foods-high-sodium.php#PWwbQuAsPORt1QDC.99

13. http://www.livestrong.com/article/296945-top-10-heart-healthy-fruits-and-vegetables/
14. http://lowfatcooking.about.com/od/lowfatbasics/a/fats1004.htm
15. http://www.nlm.nih.gov/medlineplus/ency/article/002440.htm
16. http://www.naturalnews.com/036200_asthma_diet_herbs.html#ixzz2HeX5qXLc

Chapter Ten - The King is in the Counting House
1. http://learn.bankofamerica.com/articles/managing-credit/which-credit-card-is-right-for-you.html

Finish Rich Workbook